Liam

CW01506997

anti-inflammatory

Nutrition

Heal with nutrition

Prevent illnesses

Eat well

Nutrition with

Rheumatism | Cancer

Diabetes | Gout

Autoimmune disorders

1st edition 2020

Table of contents

Dear reader!

Who is this book for? This book is for people who suffer from various health problems. As different as diseases are, they all have a common origin: subliminal inflammatory reactions. One thing is certain: the right diet is of fundamental importance to our physical condition.

This is not a diet or cookbook. It is not about renouncing all pleasure forever. The content will at least make you think, at best it will make you change your mind.

There are a number of lifestyle factors and foods that can maintain, exacerbate or trigger silent inflammation.

In this book, I will show you
- How inflammation even occurs in your body.
- Which foods cause inflammation.
- Why a plant-based, species-appropriate diet prevents inflammation.
- Which is the healthiest way to eat.

With the right nutrition, you can effectively fight inflammation and thus effectively prevent diseases. In the concept of anti-inflammatory nutrition, the preferred intake of certain unsaturated fatty acids and antioxidants plays a prominent role.

Nutrition offers everyone the chance to do something against illness, and to give the healing process a positive direction.

Best regards
Liam Wade

1. Fairytale world of healthy food

More than half of our diseases are nutritional. Statistics show that the number of chronic inflammatory diseases has increased dramatically in recent years. The trend is still upwards. The fairytale world of healthy eating fits in with this. The term "shelf life" describes the shelf life of food and beverages; how long a product can be stored without becoming unusable, or unfit for sale.

The price: poison in our food in the form of artificially produced flavors, antibacterial agents, colorings and preservatives. Responsible for this are pharmaceutical and chemical companies going hand in hand, nutrition gurus equipped with lavish consultancy contracts, unscrupulous lobbyists and politicians with the aim of creating a dream world. The advertising message: down-to-earth quality at affordable prices, produced according to granny's recipes with local ingredients from the juicy pastures of regional farmers. But this is only fantasy. The reality looks different.

In a very short time after the war, our food has been changed more than it has in the last 20,000 years. The food production industry and storage processes adapted, but not the consumers. Only and solely to the subject of economic principle, acting rationally for a specific purpose. Using given means to put the yield in relation to the market value of globally operating food companies. Well over 2,500 additives are permitted in our modern foods. But only about 300 are subject to declaration. The resuslt is an organized attack on our senses and physical integrity. Examples include hormones and antibiotics in meat, antifreeze in wine, and highly toxic ethoxyquin[1] in fish.

The food scandals of recent years have brought to light a cocktail of toxins and a trail of destruction. These include the white sausage, the intestines from China, the herbs from Poland, the veal from Hungary, Frozen bread rolls from Asia and Africa, etc. Plus plenty of phosphates and flavor enhancers. Diclofenac and sweeteners from the tap. 96% of broilers are fed with antibiotics. If one animal falls ill, the whole flock is vaccinated as a preventive measure - often even several times. This list of horrors can easily be continued page by page. The result is 25,000 deaths per year in hospitals in the European Union from multi-resistant germs. Only a few food companies provide more than 200,000 different products under an almost unmanageable number of names of retail chains.
Three out of four foods are highly industrially processed and maximized for profit.

The human evolutionary cycle of adaptation makes it impossible to adapt to this alien diet. In order to eliminate this negative development, obesity and a number of increasingly popular diseases of civilisation, this industry naturally has corresponding products in its portfolio. Dietary products, powders for shakes, colorfully and attractively packaged from the chemical building blocks of food technology - far removed from species-appropriate nutrition. Natural, fibre-rich, anti-inflammatory and nutritious food would be the focus of attention. But how can our food meet these requirements when 20% is contaminated with industrial sugar products and another 20% with white flour products? In other words, we currently cover a rounded 40% of our food intake with a maximum of carbohydrates from dead and empty food that contains vitamins, minerals and secondary plant substances only in homeopathic doses.

2. Ignition

Generally speaking, inflammation (Latin: inflammatio) is the immune system's response to an external stimulus. An inflammation is therefore part of a healing process and not a damage to the body. Inflammation is something like an early warning system—the first line of defence. Linguistically, it can be recognized by the suffix—itis. The medical term for an inflammation is usually made up of the name of the body part and the ending—itis, e.g. of the skin or appendicitis of the appendix. The aim of an inflammation is to remove the trigger, to remove harmful substances and to form replacement tissue in the course of recovery.

2.1 Causes of inflammation[2]

Inflammations have many causes. They are caused by bacteria, viruses, fungi, parasites or allergens. They can also be physical, caused by exposure to radioactive radiation or environmental toxins that overtax the immune system. With the reaction to this, the body tries to initiate a repair.

2.2 Signs of inflammation

Inflammation manifests itself in five different ways: as pain, swelling, heat, redness or in the form of a disturbed function. In the case of an insect bite, for example, we see all five signs at the same time - in the case of an eye inflammation, on the other hand, we only see redness and the leakage of tear fluid. Depending on whether the whole body or only a part of it is affected, we speak of a systemic inflammation or a local one.

2.3 Chronic inflammation

Chronic inflammation is a long-term response to inflammatory stimuli, usually accompanied by tissue injury due to the ongoing inflammatory reaction. In contrast to acute inflammatory reactions, chronic inflammation can last for weeks, months or even a lifetime in some chronic inflammatory diseases.

Many chronic inflammatory diseases begin as inferior, protracted reactions to pathogens that can act from the outside and inside. Chronic inflammation plays a key role in the development and progression of many chronic diseases e.g. autoimmune diseases, metabolic disorders such as atherosclerosis, obesity, fibrosis or cancer.

The main cause of chronic inflammation is infection—primarily, viral infections. However, stress, poor nutrition and lack of exercise also affect immune tolerance in the long term.

2.4 Silent inflammation[3]

They take the route without swelling, injury, pain or bleeding. This refers to inflammations that can be completely asymptomatic for a long time, and are not noticeable in standard blood tests. Only after a very long time will unspecific symptoms such as listlessness, loss of appetite or slight feelings of illness be noticed.

The quality of our nutrition is the counterbalance to stop chronic inflammation. White flour products, meat and sugar-rich foods are the driving force behind low-threshold inflammation. The result is an out-of-balance immune system on permanent alert. For some time now, active abdominal fat has been held responsible for the spread of inflammatory messenger substances. To get these inflammations under control, our immune system uses aggressive radicals. In the process, healthy blood vessels come into the crosshairs of the defence. This type of inflammation can appear in the brain at the first signs and seems to be partly responsible for depression. People who are slim and sporty can also be affected by silent inflammation. Environmental toxins, pesticides, preservatives, hormones in groundwater and flavor enhancers additionally damage our intestines and weaken the body's own defences.

2.5 Can inflammation be measured?

Inflamation can be measured through the following methods:

2.5.1 Blood sedimentation rate[4]

The blood sedimentation rate is a test that can be performed together with a blood test. A small amount of blood is aspirated into a very fine tube (capillary tube), which is then held upright for 3 hours. The red blood cells slowly descend in the tube. Blood components and serum separate. The speed at which this happens is measured and expressed in mm per hour. If the red blood cells sink faster than normal, this points to an an increased sedimentation rate. This occurs when the amount of proteins in the blood has increased due to disease.

2.5.2 C-reactive protein

The abbreviation CRP stands for C-reactive protein. The protein belongs to the so-called acute-phase proteins of the immune system. It is produced in the liver and distributed in the bloodstream a few hours after the inflammation. The CRP can be detected in the blood in increased amounts in the case of inflammation in the body. It is part of the immune system, and helps to remove dead immune defence cells and foreign substances from the inflamed tissue. The concentration of CRP in the blood can also provide information about the type and cause of the inflammation.

2.5.3 Fibrinogen

Fibrinogen is a protein that plays an important role in blood coagulation, and is the main factor in the plasma coagulation system. Its value is determined before operations, birth, liver diseases, thrombosis or bleeding tendency.

These methods serve as a rough guide. It is indeed possible to record success in fighting inflammation.

2.6 Less weight | less inflammation[5]

30% of the world's population is overweight. Too much weight puts enormous strain on the heart and blood circulation. The reason is: the amount of blood in obese people is greater than in that in people of normal weight. This means more work in terms of heart strain, because it has to beat more often – has high blood pressure as a consequence. Obesity also damages blood vessels in the entire organism in the long term, as deposits are encouraged, which leads to vascular calcification (arteriosclerosis).

Joint diseases and back problems are additional effects of being overweight. A person who weighs a third too much shortens his or her life expectancy by an average of 3 years - severely overweight people by up to 10 years. Visceral fat (from the Latin viscera 'the intestines') is the fat stored in the free abdominal cavity of vertebrates that envelops the internal organs, especially those of the digestive system. Thick bellies are as a result of this. The risk of diabetes and high blood pressure increases with fat deposits around the abdominal organs. There are two types of fatty tissue in our body: fat on the buttocks and hips, called subcutaneous fat and abdominal fat respectively. Subcutaneous fat tissue insulates, keeps warm and serves as an energy store for bad times. And it has one advantage: neutrality. Abdominal fat is metabolically active, primarily surrounds the liver and intestines, forms more than 200 hormone-like substances and is thus one of the largest glandular organs in humans. These messenger substances have an overall negative effect on blood pressure, insulin release and inflammation - more pronounced in men. They therefore carry a higher risk of contracting visceral fat. An abdominal girth smaller than 94cm, in women under 80cm, is considered acceptable. Stress leads to increased storage of visceral fat.

2.7 Free radicals | Antioxidants[6]

Antioxidants are nutrients that help to minimize the damage free radicals cause to the body. Free radicals are highly reactive compounds that are formed during normal metabolic functions in the body or released from the environment, for example, through exposure to pollution and other toxins. Unstable free radicals contain "extra" energy that they try to reduce by reacting with chemicals in the body, which impairs the normal functioning of cells. Antioxidants fight free radicals in several ways: They can reduce free radical energy, stop free radical formation, or interrupt an oxidizing chain reaction to minimize the damage caused by free radicals.

Consuming a variety of antioxidant enzymes, vitamins, minerals and herbs can be the best way to comprehensively protect our bodies from free radical damage.

In addition to enzymes, many vitamins and minerals act as independent antioxidants such as vitamin C, vitamin E, beta-carotene, lutein, lycopene, vitamin B2, coenzyme Q10 and cysteine (an amino acid). Herbs or berries such as blueberries, turmeric, grape seed or pine bark extracts and ginkgo can provide strong antioxidant protection for the body.

Free radicals are believed to play a role in more than 60 different health conditions, including aging, cancer and atherosclerosis. Reducing the vulnerability to free radicals and increasing the absorption of antioxidant nutrients can reduce the risk of free radical-related health problems.

2.8 Anti-inflammable food
2.8.1 Wholemeal products

The fibre in wholemeal products aids digestion, helps to lower blood fat levels and slows down the rise in blood sugar. In addition, numerous studies show that a wholemeal diet can significantly reduce the risk of heart attack, stroke and type 2 diabetes. In addition, they are real miracle weapons against abdominal fat, which is metabolically active and therefore promotes inflammation. Omega 3 fatty acids

2.8.2 Nuts | Seeds | Vegetable oils

Seeds and nuts contain valuable fibre, as well as antioxidant minerals such as magnesium, selenium and zinc. Walnuts are also rich in Omega 3 fatty acids, which have anti-inflammatory effects. Hemp oil, linseed oil, wheat germ oil and coconut oil are also particularly recommended due to their high accumulation of omega 3 fatty acids, vitamin A and vitamin B. Due to the high concentration of omega 6 fatty acids, sunflower seed oil, safflower oil, peanut oil, corn germ oil and sunflower oil are not recommended.

2.8.3 Omega 3 fatty acids[7]

Foods high in Omega 3 include fatty sea fish such as salmon, mackerel and anchovies. Walnuts and linseed also have a high proportion of Omega 3 fatty acids. With omega 3 rich vegetable oils, care should be taken not to heat them up too high and consume them quickly.

2.8.4 Purple, blue, red fruits and vegetables

Polyphenols, resveratrol, flavonoids and anthocyanins7 are found in the marginal layers of leaves and plants. Anthocyanins, which belong to the flavonoids, contain many healthy active substances. The potent antioxidants have antiviral, anti-inflammatory and anti-cancer effects, for example. The fruits and vegetables in question are berries, pomegranates, plums and beetroot. The above mentioned ingredients are also contained in many spices as well as red wine and cocoa.

2.8.5 Herbs and spices

Many herbs and spices contain numerous ingredients with anti-inflammatory properties. This is due to the essential oils. Wild garlic, for example, contains many essential oils- vitamin C, mustard oil glycosides and flavonoids. Nutritional science knows of several thousand compounds of these secondary plant substances, which are classified into subgroups such as flavones, flavanols, flavana or flavanones. Basil shines through essential oil, terpenes and flavonoids - savory through tanning agents.

2.8.6 Onions and garlic

The sulphur-containing compound (a sulphide called allicin), which causes an odor and is not appreciated by everyone, has a positive effect on health. The secondary plant compounds not only provide an intense odor during processing, they are also antibiotic, blood pressure and cholesterol-lowering.

2.9 Inflammatory foods[8]
2.9.1 Sugar

Sugar is a dose of dependent poison. One in five sugar consumers is considered obese. In the last 100 years, the per capita consumption of sugar in this country has risen by a factor of 50, causing a whole range of serious diseases. Sugar is a trigger for inflammation in our body.

2.9.1.1 Metabolic syndrome[9]

The metabolic syndrome is a generic term for various disorders caused by excessive sugar consumption. The Greek term "metabolic" means metabolism related. One speaks of a syndrome when different symptoms occur at the same time (complex symptoms), each of which can have a different trigger.

2.9.1.2 Type 2 diabetes

Everyday, more than 1000 persons are diagnosed with type 2 diabetes, a total of more than 7.5 million. The disease affects younger people more often. Many think they are healthy and only feel a little flabby now and then. There can be many reasons why they may be ill, but only very few of them come up with that. At first, diabetes does not cause any complaints worth mentioning or even none at all; these only occur when blood sugar is elevated.

If we have too much sugar in our blood, our body does not report this. The warning signal pain does not manifest in this case. None of those affected will notice at first that a disease is imminent. Before an operation or a control examination, it is usually recognized by chance that the sugar level is elevated and thus diabetes. Only when the blood sugar level is permanently too high do doctors speak of diabetes type 2. At the beginning of the disease, the pancreas produces too much insulin to ensure that the sugar reaches the cells after all. Doctors suspect that sooner or later the insulin-producing cells are overstrained and can no longer produce insulin. Damage to the heart, kidneys, eyes and veins is caused by sugar circulating in the bloodstream. The risk of a stroke or heart attack is up to four times higher in persons with this disease.

The cost of type 2 diabetes is estimated to be about 21 billion / year. Diabetes and secondary diseases are an enormous burden on the health care system, and a major threat to the mental and physical health of those affected. Diabetes type 2 is reversible and therefore curable. Provided we reduce our sugar consumption, lose weight and get more exercise.

2.9.1.3 Heredity and lifestyle

The vast majority of people with diabetes are people with type 2 diabetes. 15-22% of people over 65 years of age have diabetes, comprising more men than women. If you have passed the age of 70, there are more women than men.

Whether a person has type 2 diabetes is dependent on lifestyle and heredity. Anyone with a predisposition for type 2 diabetes can counteract the disease by taking plenty of exercise and eating appropriate food. Studies have shown that 50% of these people did not become diabetic. It is recommended that blood sugar levels be checked regularly by doctors.

2.9.1.4 Symptoms

It often takes several years before type 2 diabetes is detected – the warning signals are not clear. Nevertheless, there are indications where you should listen carefully. For example, you may feel a bit tired, need to sleep a lot or are constantly thirsty and often have to go to the toilet. You lose weight for no reason - the skin on your feet is unusually dry.

2.9.1.5 Destroyed nerves

Diabetes type 2 sufferers are often diagnosed with a visual impairment. Many find it difficult to see at close range. If there is too much sugar in the blood, the nerves are attacked. One in ten patients complain of neuropathic pain, a nerve damage.

The fingertips start to tingle and the sensitivity of the feet diminishes. There are often digestive problems, and some patients complain of flatulence, constipation, diarrhoea or abdominal pain.

2.9.1.6 Forms of diabetes

The manifestations of diabetes are different—the following is a detailed description.

Type 1: Less than 10% of diabetes patients are victims of this type. The immune system of these people is affected by a malfunction. The cells responsible for insulin have been destroyed during this process. Too little insulin is produced. There is no cure for this type of diabetes.

Type 2: Unlike type 1, type 2 is not a disease of the immune system, but is caused by lifestyle mistakes. 90%

of diabetes patients are affected. In contrast to type 1, this type is curable.

Gestational diabetes: During pregnancy, the placenta produces many more hormones so that the baby can develop properly. However, these pregnancy hormones can interfere with the action of insulin. The pancreas therefore releases more insulin to supply cells and tissue. This process takes place mainly in the second half of pregnancy. Some pregnant women have problems, so glucose is not absorbed by the cells but accumulates in the blood. From this point on, one speaks of gestational diabetes. Normally the blood sugar level returns to normal shortly after delivery. If gestational diabetes is not detected, this can have serious consequences for mother and child.

Type 3: Here you will find all types of diabetes that cannot be classified into type 1 and type 2. The cause can be a viral infection, a genetic mutation, or damage to the pancreas.

2.9.1.7 Is sugar addictive?
Definite answer: yes. Addiction doesn't happen overnight. It usually sneaks into life unnoticed. Because it's not uncommon to eat a piece of chocolate. At first it's no problem. Or is it?

Addiction requires a susceptible brain and other factors. Alcohol, nicotine, or in this case sugar, are the foundations of addiction.

The scientific explanation: The balance of serotonin and dopamine in the brain is disturbed. If the messenger substance serotonin is too low and the dopamine level is too high at the same time, or if both substances are present in insufficient concentrations, the basic conditions are present for becoming addicted.

Dopamine is a largely excitatory nerve transmitter of the central nervous system and is used for communication. It is released in the brain when we are full of anticipation, for example before a romantic meeting, a competition or a hoped-for sense of achievement. It conveys a positive emotional experience and is also called the happiness hormone. If there is the first kiss or exceptional praise from the boss, serotonin is released. This messenger substance stands for happiness, satisfaction, relaxation and satisfaction.

If the dopamine level drops, we suffer from lack of drive and inertia. If we are moody, disappointed and worried, this has to do with serotonin deficiency and in such a state we reach for the drug sugar which we know. This increases dopamine and serotonin levels and gives us a feeling of happiness and relaxation. They pretend to us humans that we have achieved something extraordinary. Now, let's talk about the scientific background.

The sugar industry has long denied that there is such a thing as addiction in connection with sugar. However, there is clear scientific evidence. The enormous potential for addiction has been demonstrated in rats, among other things. When rats accustomed to sugar are deprived of their daily dose, they react with trembling, chattering teeth and fear. The rats then increasingly use alcohol as a substitute. When sugar was on the menu, however, they ate more than ever before. Humans show very similar patterns of behavior.

After only a short time, changes in the brain of the rats similar to those found in chronic drug addicts were diagnosed. Drugs and alcohol addicts have a conspicuous weakness for sugar products. Sugar is the number one popular drug.

Conclusion: Sugar acts like alcohol and nicotine, increases serotonin and dopamine levels, can be called a drug and will lead to addiction if consumed in excess.

2.9.1.8 Does sugar cause cancer?

This thesis is considered to be unsubstantiated, but there is clear evidence to support it. A Belgian research team found in a nine-year study that sugar stimulates tumor growth. In the study, the scientists observed the so-called Warburg effect over a long period of time. This mechanism, which has been known for a long time, shows in the laboratory that cancer cells metabolise larger amounts of sugar than healthy cells.

The Canadian anthropologist Vilhjámur Stefánsson observed something astonishing at the beginning of the 20th century: Eskimos did not get cancer as long as they ate the traditional diet. They went hunting, kept to fixed daily rhythms, ate meat from seals, caribou or fish. It was only when they switched to carbohydrate-rich industrial food in the middle of the 20th century and became somewhat more comfortable that they died of cancer.

2.9.2 Trans fats[10]

2.9.2.1 Properties Trans fatty acids

Natural unprocessed foods contain two types of fatty acids - saturated and unsaturated. Saturated fatty acids, which come from animal fats (meat, lard, dairy products) and tropical oils such as coconut or palm oil, can increase the LDL cholesterol (bad cholesterol) level in the blood.

Unsaturated fatty acids generally do not raise or lower cholesterol levels.

Trans fats are the third form of fatty acids. Trans fats are unsaturated fatty acids which are artificially industrially hardened and which our body cannot process. This happens e.g. to make vegetable oils spreadable. While trans fats are found in minute amounts in a few foods (especially dairy products and meat from cows and sheep), almost all trans fats currently in our diet come from an industrial process in which unsaturated fatty acids from vegetable oil are added hydrogen.

However, unsaturated fatty acids are also formed during multiple strong heating and frying of unsaturated fatty acids, e.g. in deep fryers. In the process, molecular structures are changed. The advantage of trans fats for the food industry is that cheap vegetable oils can be solidified and stabilised. As they are available in solid form instead of liquid form, trans fats can be used as a substitute for saturated fats in food to extend the shelf life.

2.9.2.2 Health impact

The World Health Organization wants to ban these fats because they play a role in the development of heart attacks and strokes. This has already been done in

America. Trans fats cause an increased level of LDL cholesterol in the blood. Low density lipoprotein (LDL) transports fat from the liver into body cells. Once the cholesterol requirement is met, residual cholesterol remains in the blood, which leads to rising cholesterol levels. Too much cholesterol in the blood is dangerous. Crystals can form and deposit on the walls of the arteries. The body's own defence system reacts to the sharp-edged coating with inflammation in the vessel wall - atherosclerotic plaques form, which constrict blood vessels.

2.9.3 Meat consumption

The anti-inflammatory effect of plant foods is more than just the power of plants. It is the avoidance of animal products. A single meal of meat, dairy products and eggs triggers an inflammatory reaction in the body within hours of consumption. A whole range of diseases including osteoarthritis, diabetes, rheumatism and colon cancer are the result of excessive meat consumption. The reason: the intestinal environment and with it the microbiome is affected. Potentially aggressive bacteria are on the rise and in the long term cause inflammation and intestinal cancer. The World Health Organization has already drawn the consequences by 2015. Red and processed meat has been considered safe for carcinogenicity since then. A similar risk level is now only assigned to nicotine.

2.9.4 White flour products

Pronounced consumption of white flour products leads to the proliferation of inflammatory intestinal bacteria. Wholemeal products, on the other hand, have a number of positive side effects such as minerals and fibre. They are metabolized much more slowly, which leads to a constant increase in blood sugar levels and a slow release of insulin. Attacks of ravenous hunger remain the rarity. White flour products have the same effect as sugar.

2.9.5 Alcohol consumption

The plasma protein CRP is part of the body's own defence system. The amount of CRP in the blood increases significantly if people drink too much alcohol over a longer period of time. The level of CRP in the blood also rises in the case of infections, inflammations and tissue damage. An elevated CRP level does not allow a conclusion to be drawn about a specific disease, but requires further diagnostic measures. In addition, a whole range of massively harmful effects of alcohol consumption are probably known.

2.9.6 Omega 6 fatty acids

Omega-6 fatty acids act as components of the cell membrane— are needed for growth and repair processes, and are the natural antagonists of omega-3 fatty acids. The body can also produce tissue hormones from arachidonic acid - the eicosanoids. They promote inflammation as part of the immune system. Basically a healthy condition. However, the proportion of omega 6 fatty acids in our food intake is at least 15 times too high. Meat from factory farming has a particularly high content of Omega 6 fatty acids. Vegetable tops are soya oil, sunflower oil and margarine.

2.9.7 Milk | Milk products

There are quite a few people who suffer from joint and bone pain after eating dairy products. The trigger: the casein contained in many dairy products. This is a cocktail of proteins that make up about ¾ of the total amount of proteins in milk. Milk has a biological mission. Signalling substances in milk, which are intended for babies and children, stimulate growth and are exactly what is needed here.

For adults, however, this can be dangerous. Large quantities of milk stimulate the hormone "insulin-like growth factor 1", or IGF-1 for short. It promotes cell growth, including that of tumour cells. Fresh milk contains the amino acids valine, isoleucine and lecithin, which are growth-promoting gene messengers. By consuming cow's milk, the consumer takes in about 250 messenger substances that can have an effect on over 10,000 human genes. Overweight, diabetes risk, cancer and unnatural tissue growth are associated with this.

2.10 Immune System

The immune system is active at all human interfaces with the outside world. If there is a confrontation by viruses, fungal spores, bacteria or other environmental toxins, our immune shield comes into play. The largest of these is the intestinal immune system. It reacts to "old enemies", which are mainly found in nature. This is what it is designed for. Mechanisms developed over thousands of years, e.g. vomiting, nausea or diarrhoea, are supposed to prevent the deeper penetration of pathogenic toxins. Inflammations of the eyes, sinuses or ears can be typical initial reactions of this safety device. Inflammations are the body's own means to solve problems. Mantra-like statements by the pharmaceutical industry that inflammations must be contained or even prevented are often aimed solely at the sales results of various drugs that can be purchased in pharmacies.

2.11 Bowel Health[11]

It is estimated that the human gastrointestinal tract is colonized by an amount of 10 to the power of 14 bacteria, which would be about 10 times the total number of cells in the human body. A disturbance of the intestinal flora is associated with severe physical defects, including metabolic diseases, cancer and autoimmune diseases. Researchers assume that currently 1-10% of intestinal bacteria are known and studied.

2.11.1 What makes the intestine so unique?

When it causes complaints, some people first realize how important our intestines are. In recent years, it has increasingly come into focus because it is very likely to play a central role in the development of a variety of diseases. For more than 10 years now, the intestinal bacteria have been increasingly on the trail and it has been noticed that many diseases are accompanied by a disturbance of the intestinal flora. Its length is about 8 meters, its diameter a few centimeters. More remarkable is the surface of 30 to 40 square meters. It is therefore the largest contact surface between us and the outside world. Inside the intestinal anatomy, a myriad of intestinal villi are responsible for this fact. Meals need up to 3 days to pass through the intestine. This organ acts completely independently; It perceives, corrects, learns and is the seat of intuition. The enteric nervous system (ENS) enables the intestine to function as the only organ independent of the central nervous system (CNS). The brain contains around 100 billion neurons, the number in the ENS is estimated at 100 to 200 million. The ENS is structurally and functionally similar to the brain. The intestine essentially performs two tasks. The food taken in through the mouth reaches the large intestine via the stomach and small intestine. There, vital substances are extracted from the nutrient slurry and supplied to our body. For intruders such as poisons, viruses, toxins, fungi or other pathogens, the journey normally ends at this point in a healthy intestine.

The intestine is therefore the largest defence and immune system of our body. More than 70% of the defence and immune system is located in the intestine. Several hundred trillion intestinal bacteria and microorganisms have colonised our intestines. More microorganisms live in one gram of intestinal bacteria than people on earth. The constitution and composition of these bacteria are largely responsible for our health and well-being.

The intestine in cooperation with the brain decides which food components are metabolised if, how and when. These microorganisms have a decisive influence on whether we remain healthy or are susceptible to disease. Equally positive for intestinal health: avoid stress and regularly ensure sufficient sleep. People who sleep less than 6 hours on the average have an increased risk of bowel cancer. Diets rich in fibre, such as pulses, plenty of fresh vegetables and fruit and wholemeal products, strengthen the functions of the bowel.

2.11.2 Intestinal bacteria

A distinction is made between coliform bacteria, the bad intestinal bacteria, and probiotics, the good intestinal bacteria. E. coli bacteria produce toxic substances such as indole and skatole when they break down protein. The more odorless our urine, sweat and stools are, the more smoothly our detoxification and digestive system functions.

2.11.2.1 Good gut bacteria

The good intestinal bacteria help to protect us by displacing some of their dangerous relatives that can cause disease and are therefore the natural antagonists of E. coli bacteria. They keep the intestinal environment in balance. They should have a percentage of over 85 percent. Good bacteria are used in medicine to produce antibiotics or in food production to make fermented foods, such as sauerkraut, yoghurt, kimchi and kombucha. The two best known of their kind are Lactobacillus acidophilus and Bifidobacterium bifidus. These primarily produce acetic acid, lactic acid, digestive enzymes and vitamins.

2.11.2.2 Bad intestinal bacteria

Every individual carries bad intestinal bacteria in addition to the good gut bacteria. They are called pathogenic because they cause infections, make us ill and in rare cases can be fatal. Bad bacteria are caused by external influences such as food, environmental toxins or the effects of stress on our body. Too many antibiotics, excessively misplaced hygiene, improperly prepared food, too much sugar in our food, stress and lack of sleep are some of the things that can lead to a sick intestinal flora.

3. Nutrition

3.1 Nutrition in the course of time

Apart from a few exceptions, man and his ancestors have, during most of the history of development, eaten mainly or exclusively vegetable food. This is evidenced by anatomical peculiarities such as the inability of humans to synthesize vitamin C and the lack of an enzyme that breaks down uric acid. Some researchers have even described the human dentition as that of a fructifier, and the structure of the colon also corresponds to that of a herbivore.

Nowadays, a diet rich in meat can have unhealthy consequences because our lifestyle have changed fundamentally. In the past, meat came from free range animals whose feed was not industrial waste. Food had to be hunted and earned and was associated with hard physical work.

3.2 Food of our ancestors

- was free of sugar.
- was rich in secondary plant compounds.
- was rich in fiber.
- was species-appropriate.
- consisted of whole grains.
- had a balanced ratio of Omega 3 to Omega 6 fatty acids.

- was predominantly vegetable and had few animal components.

3.3 Nutrition of today

- has a very long list of additives such as baking agents, preservatives, colorants, synthetically produced flavors, emulsifiers, etc.
- contains a high proportion of animal meat and sausage products, which also originate from factory farming.
- has a sugar concentration increased by a factor of 50 since the last 100 years in almost all industrially produced food.
- accepts damage to the intestinal flora caused by medication.
- has a much too low consumption of drinking water of spring water quality.
- means irradiation of food.
- is a system that has been proven to be contaminated by fungicides and pesticides.

3.4 What is healthy body weight?

People with a few kilos too much are often pigeonholed as "sick" and "lazy". The weight alone does not make any statement about the state of health. Many people try to counteract the common weight norms and develop a positive relationship with their body. According to sociologists, if you are slim, you avoid having a certain amount of capital that you can exchange for friendship, partnership or professional success. Slim people, according to sociologists, are unconsciously perceived as more trustworthy, competent, successful and healthy, unlike those whose appearance is rather below the norm. Unjust but probably human. Because we humans like things to be simple. At this point, however, the only question that interests us is what healthy weight can be.

Measurement methods for a healthy body weight
Many have an individual feel-good weight - but health risks due to too many or too few pounds on the ribs can be estimated quite accurately. Body Mass Index (BMI) and Waist-Hip-Ratio (WHtR) show quickly and easily whether you are normal, underweight or overweight: if you are significantly overweight, just 5% less body fat will lower your blood pressure and improve your blood lipid levels.

Calculate BMI19 (Body Mass Index)

The Body Mass Index is the most commonly used value for assessing body weight—it helps you to better estimate your weight. It puts your body weight in relation to your height. More precisely, the body weight in kilograms is related to the height in metres squared. Important to know: the Body Mass Index allows only a first rough estimate. For example, someone who has a lot of muscle mass can have a high BMI without being overweight in the true sense of the word. The BMI also says nothing about the distribution of body fat. In particular, too much belly fat is considered a health risk. Different rules apply to children, as they are still growing. There are special BMI tables for them.

Example: You are 1.70 metres tall and weigh 80 kilograms. Then you do the math:

1.70 x 1.70 = 2.89 now divide your weight by this value: 80 / 2.89 = 27.7

27.7 - or rounded up 28—is your body mass index.

Rate BMI (Body Mass Index)
The ideal BMI value for women is between 19 and 24, for men between 20 and 25, which statistically is the highest BMI value for life expectancy. However, the ideal BMI is

also dependent on age. And it is by no means the measure of all things.

BMI classification of the World Health Organization (WHO):

Category	male	female
Underweight	less than 20	less than 19
Normal weight	20-24.9	19-23.9
Overweight	25-29.9	24-29.9
massive overweight (Grade I obesity)	30-34.9	30-34.9
Obesity grade II	35-39.9	35-39.9
Obesity grade III	40 or more	40 or more

Calculate WHtR (waist-hip quotient)

Many experts therefore consider the value "waist circumference in centimeters divided by height in centimeters" (Waist-to-Height-Ratio, abbreviated WHtR) to be more meaningful. Here, a value below 0.5 (for older people below 0.6) is considered desirable. The waist circumference alone also helps for rough orientation: it should not be more than 102 centimetres for men and 88 centimetres for women.

Rate WHtR (waist-hip quotient)

Measure the waist circumference between the lowest ribcage and the iliac crest. For the hip circumference, find the longest distance around your buttocks.

Example: A woman on an empty stomach has 71cm waist circumference and 95cm hip circumference.

The WHtR is therefore: 71cm ÷ 95cm = 0.75cm

For people of average height, the waist or abdominal circumference can provide information about existing obesity. WHtR values (and waist circumference) of adult women and men are defined as follows.

Women:
Normal weight WHtR > 0.85 Waist circumference > 80cm
Overweight WHtR < 0.85 Waist circumference 80 to 87.9cm
Adiposity WHtR from 0.85 waist circumference over 88cm

Men:
Normal weight WHtR > 1.0 Waist circumference > 94cm
Overweight WHtR < 1.0 Waist circumference 94 to 101.9cm
Adiposity WHtR from 1.0 waist circumference over 102cm

3.5 Balanced nutrition

The so-called Mediterranean Diet is widely recommended by medical professionals. It was voted the best form of nutrition in 2019. The main ingredients are fish, olive oil, nuts, salad and fresh vegetables. Fatty milk and red meat in large quantities are taboo. This form of nutrition helps you to reach your desired weight. High blood pressure and cardiovascular diseases are the result of too much salt in our diet, which is often the case with ready-made foods.

• Do not buy a product for which advertising is made because they are highly processed and therefore harmful in every respect.

• Avoid sweetened drinks and drink only water, tea or coffee pure. Sugar is often used as a cheap filler and flavor enhancer in convenience foods. If you cook for yourself, you know what's in the food.

• Getting to know and appreciate natural sweetness again - like in natural fruit, primarily berries. These have a low sugar content (about 4-8g carbohydrates per 100g) and are also packed full of nutrients and antioxidants. There is nothing wrong with berries. They are even recommended due to their nutrient profile.

However, it is always important to keep an eye on the exact amount.

• Try to eat fresh food as much as possible and do not eat ready-made meals, which often contain sugar. In any case plenty of vegetables and salad.

• Those who start their meals with salads, vegetables and protein-rich foods, and only then switch to carbohydrate-rich foods, eat healthier, because the blood sugar level and thus the insulin secretion remain lower than if you eat the same food in reverse order. Avoid eating carbohydrate-rich foods such as rice, potatoes, pasta, bread or even sweets on an empty stomach. It is not for nothing that a dessert is always at the end of a menu.

• Appetite is curbed by bitter substances. Chewing the bitter calamus root is an old household remedy for ravenous appetite. You can make a tea from it. Chocolate with 70-90% cocoa content tastes bitter and prevents the greed for sweets. Coffee with its bitter substances is also a good appetite suppressant. In the evening, it is better to drink decaffeinated coffee.

• Herbs like coriander, thyme, parsley and wild garlic replace salt. This also includes the use of garlic and onions. Sweets should be compensated for by eating nuts, which contain a high proportion of fibre and protein, as a healthy snack. Red meat is on the menu of Mediterranean cuisine twice a week at most. Instead, poultry and fish are used as a source of protein. Milk in the high-fat version should be replaced by consistent use of low-fat milk. Fruits and vegetables are eaten throughout the day and are the primary ingredients. It is of central importance to "take your time" and to enjoy while eating and to chew slowly. The speed at which one eats food has a considerable influence on the storage of depot fat.

3.6 Why a high fibre diet?

Fibre stimulates digestion and prevents various diseases. Studies have shown that a lack of fibre is a risk factor for overweight, diabetes, high blood pressure, heart attack and other complaints. With a diet rich in fibre you can lose weight very well. This is because fibre has the property of bloating in the intestines. This suggests to our body that we are full and promotes the feeling of satiety.

3.6.1 What are dietary fibres?

Dietary fibres are vegetable fibres and swelling agents and largely indigestible food components, mostly carbohydrates, which are mainly found in vegetable foods. They are mainly found in cereals, fruit, vegetables, legumes and, in small quantities, in milk. For the sake of simplicity, fibre is divided into water-soluble (such as locust bean gum, guar, pectin and dextrins) and water-insoluble (for example cellulose). Dietary fibres are, quite contrary to what the name suggests, an important part of the human diet. Their energy value is 8 kJ/g.

3.6.2 Effects of fibres

Water-insoluble dietary fibres (such as cellulose, lignin) are source material and provide "mass". In combination with sufficient liquid, they swell up in the stomach and thus make you full. They also accelerate the intestinal passage. They "clean" the intestine like a sponge.

Water-soluble dietary fibres (for example pectin, inulin, oligofructose and other prebiotics) are "bacterial food". They nourish our intestinal flora. These microorganisms are vital. They help us to utilize our food and produce the healthy short-chain fatty acids.

Water-soluble dietary fibres have a positive effect on:
- the sugar metabolism.
- the fat metabolism.
- the regulation of the immune system.
- the nervous system.

Beta-glucans, soluble fibres in oats and barley, are particularly good for diabetics; they can intercept blood sugar peaks and counteract insulin resistance.

3.6.3 How many grams of fibre does the body need?

You should consume between 30 and 40 grams of fibre a day. 15-20g should come from cereals and cereal products, the rest in the form of vegetables, fruit, nuts and pulses.

3.6.4 What should be considered with dietary fibres?

Fibre swells up in the intestines. This means that the intestinal volume increases significantly. In order to swell and to stimulate intestinal activity, your intestine needs fluid. The recommended amount to drink is 4% of your body weight.

3.7 Fasting | Impulse for self-healing

Fasting as an integral part of nutritional medicine, is considered a multi-talent and has a number of drastic advantages. Under consideration of anti-inflammatory nutrition I would like to deal here exclusively with interval fasting.

3.7.1 Autophagy | Ketosis

In order to live, our body needs energy, which it generates with the help of the basic building blocks contained in food. This produces valuable and not so valuable substances, some of which are harmful to humans and then leave the body through detoxification processes.

Autophagy is derived from the Greek word "car" for self and "phagia" for food. In 2016, the subject became more popular as the Japanese Yoshiori Ohsumi was awarded a Nobel Prize in Medicine for his research on the subject. Autophagy is our body's recycling program, in which cellular waste is identified, recycled or excreted through the skin, lungs, blood and urine. If this program fails, the consequences include neurodegenerative diseases such as Alzheimer's, Parkinson's, cancer or increased susceptibility to infection.

Our body has several sources for generating energy. The first source is called sugar (carbohydrates or glucose), the second is fat. Glucose is stored in the liver and muscles. This storage is empty after 24-72 hours under normal stress. Our brain is exclusively dependent on glucose and cannot use protein or fat. For this reason, we are able to produce alternative energy sources, the so-called ketone bodies, which are formed from fatty acids. The formation of ketone bodies from fat is possible for up to 60 days. After that, these reserves are also used up. This period of time is called ketosis or hunger metabolism. In order to reach this state outside of famines, it is necessary to reduce the intake of glucose / sugar / carbohydrates to a maximum of about 20g per day.

3.7.2 Interval Fasting

Interval fasting, also known as intermittent fasting, is particularly concerned with the time of food intake, for which there are different variants. This flexibility makes it possible to find the right method for individual needs. Three forms are particularly popular.

Method 16:8:

In this method, no food is eaten for 16 hours straight. During the remaining eight hours of the day you can eat as usual. During this time a balanced diet is recommended. It can be decided individually whether breakfast is omitted or dinner is eaten during the 16 hour fast.

Method 5:2:

Five days a week you eat as usual, on two days you reduce your calorie intake to a minimum. Women then consume about 500kcal, men 600kcal. The fasting days do not have to follow each other and can vary from week to week. Here, fasting is done every second day and the calorie intake is minimised to 500kcal for women and 600kcal for men.

Interval fasting attacks so-called visceral fat. This fat accumulates in the middle of the body and is suspected to produce and distribute hormones and inflammatory substances like an independent organ. In most people the hormonal balance is disturbed. Every intake of calories boosts the release of insulin and thus activates the storage of nutrients. With the release of insulin, a decrease in body fat is impossible. Insulin is used in factory farming specifically to build weight. The "hunger hormone" ghrelin is inhibited and thus ensures a feeling of satiety. Once fat is converted into ketone body, it is either consumed or excreted in the urine. Ketone bodies are not stored temporarily.

3.7.2.1 What interval fasting still achieves

Oxidative stress and inflammation

Oxidative stress is triggered by free radicals. In our body there must be a harmony between oxidants and antioxidants. Free radicals are intermediate products of our metabolism. They are oxygen compounds that lack an electron. If the body does not succeed in restoring the balance, inflammations arise. Interval fasting helps you to establish this harmony, especially by removing free radicals in times of ketosis.

Aging

Interval fasting slows down aging. By lowering blood sugar, strengthening the immune system, improving cell regeneration and reducing blood pressure, the aging process is delayed. The basis for this is autophagy and ketosis.

Sleep

Unhealthy and late eating means detrimental sleep. Those who eat too late and especially before going to bed provide little or no rest at night. Interval fasting regulates the biorhythm and thus prevents a negative sleep experience or contributes to improvement.

Metabolism

The metabolism is changed from food from outside to food from inside. Interval fasting promotes the process of glycogenosis. This is the conversion of glucose to glycogen. Urea is synthesized as a by-product. This is excreted through the kidneys. Liver and kidney are relieved overall.

Increase of the inner focus

Due to the increased and altered supply of energy in ketosis, the brain works better and more effectively. As an early remedy for epilepsy it led to massive improvements and stabilization of the patients.

Somatic cells

During autophagy, the renewal of body cells and organs is much faster and more flexible. Interval fasting controls and reprogrammes liver proteins and thus has a direct effect on liver health. The metabolism of fatty acids is also positively influenced.

Depressions

It has been known for a long time that short food deprivation increases the tryptophan levels in the brain. L-Tryptophan belongs to the 21 proteinogenic amino acids, those that are needed for the body's own protein synthesis.

A low tryptophan level can lead to reduced memory performance. Various general conditions such as unhealthy nutrition or stress have a negative influence on the tryptophan level in our body.

Digestion and intestinal flora

During interval fasting the acid-base balance is regulated. Flour, coffee, sugary foods and alcohol, among other factors, cause the intestinal flora to be impaired and not get the chance to regenerate. The intestine contains 80% of the immune system. Bacteria in the intestine provide metabolic products. They influence our immune system and can moderate or promote inflammatory processes.

Favourably influencing cancer diseases

There is much evidence that intermittent fasting can prevent cancer or even have a positive effect on advanced stages of the disease.

You have open questions or concerns? - write me a mail to book_manufacture@outlook.com.

3.8 Alkaline diet

A whole range of health and nutrition experts consider the overacidification of the organism to be the cause of various complaints. They believe that, for example, the typically meat-rich western diet, which is based on an excess of animal ingredients, is responsible for more acids in the body. Basic foods such as vegetables are not consumed in sufficient quantities. In addition, buffer substances such as minerals, for example calcium or magnesium, are lacking. In this situation, our body is not able to excrete excess acids through the lungs, kidneys, intestines and sweat. Every cell in our body functions best within a certain pH range. This zone defines whether something is acidic, neutral or alkaline. A pH value below 7 indicates that something is acidic, a pH value above 7 indicates that something is alkaline. Blood is in the slightly alkaline range with 7.35 to 7.44. Many organs function best in a certain pH range. Therefore, humans are constantly busy maintaining this ideal range and buffering and balancing acids. Our body permanently deacidifies. With nutrition and some small changes, you can help restore your balance.

3.8.1 Seven steps acid bases household

• **Most important factor: nutrition.** Alkaline foods are rich in minerals because they buffer the acids in the body. This includes vegetables, especially green leafy vegetables such as spinach. Herbs such as nettle or dandelion are also included. The taste of a food does not indicate whether it is metabolized to form acids or bases. Fruit acids from oranges and lemons are metabolized in our body to form bases.

• **Reduce acid-forming foods to a minimum.** These foods contain mainly sulphur-containing amino acids. These include meat, fish, cheese and eggs. Whole grain products and legumes are also acidogenic, but they contain important nutrients and are good acid producers. Sweets and baked goods made from white flour should be avoided.

• **Pay attention to your breathing and avoid shallow breathing.** The lungs are an important organ that helps with deacidification. Acids in the body are converted to carbon dioxide in the lungs and breathed out. The more intensively you breathe, the better your body is supported in the deacidification process.

• **Support the liver and kidney during deacidification.** Both are important organs that help your body eliminate acids. Drinking enough water is absolutely necessary. Water enriched with lemon juice is best suited. Avoid alcohol, as it acts as a cell poison and restricts liver activity.

• **If you implement these advices more than 80%, you have** already achieved a lot. This procedure is called base excess nutrition. The remaining 20% should be covered by good acid producers like fish.

• **Pay attention to skin care.** Therefore regular sweating is advisable when visiting the sauna or doing sports.

- **Stress is avoided** because it leads to reduced activity of liver, kidneys and intestines. In addition, breathing is not sufficiently deep.

3.9 Fermented food

Yoghurt, cheese, kefir, wine, beer and sauerkraut all have one thing in common; they are preserved by fermentation. Used for thousands of years. Healthy nutrients and a long shelf life—that's the promise of food fermentation. Beverages, vegetables and co. are packed in preserving jars and left to ferment in a brine. In the process, they develop valuable probiotic substances, lactic acid bacteria, the pH value changes and they become durable. Ferments are free of preservatives and additives, healthy and tasty. This type of food contains natural enzymes, creates a positive environment in the intestines by consuming lactic acid bacteria, and thus strengthens our immune system. Since 70% to 80% of the immune system is located in the intestine, the right balance of the intestinal flora, as you have already known, is important. A high vitamin content and secondary plant substances have an antioxidant, immunostimulating and anticoagulant effect. They can thus positively counteract cancer, diabetes and cardiovascular diseases. A further effect: regular consumption of fermented food can prevent ravenous appetite, as there are fewer harmful microorganisms in the intestine. This in turn is important to ensure that the metabolism runs smoothly and that all the nutrients important to the body can be absorbed.

In the late 19th century it was recognized that microorganisms in the gastrointestinal tract of healthy people were different from that of those who were ill. This beneficial flora was called probiotics, which literally means "for life". Probiotics are microorganisms that have been proven to have beneficial effects on health.

Fermentation helps to form new nutrients such as B vitamins, folic acid, riboflavin, niacin, thiamine and biotin and has been shown to improve the availability, digestibility and quantity of some nutrients.

3.9.1 Overview fermented food

Sauerkraut

Sauerkraut is not a separate plant or cabbage genus, but is the name given to cabbage preserved by lactic fermentation. The most common types of cabbage are white cabbage and pointed cabbage. To turn cabbage into sauerkraut, all that is needed is a little salt and time. The rest is taken care of by the lactic acid bacteria that form on their own. The importance of sauerkraut for the diet grew especially in Central and Eastern Europe in areas with long, cold winters. People realised that sauerkraut's shelf life and high vitamin content made it ideal for protecting them from deficiency symptoms during the winter. At the same time, it could be produced and stored relatively easily and without great effort.

Yoghurt

Yoghurt originally comes from the Balkans. There it was not made from cow's milk, but from goat, sheep and buffalo milk. Yoghurt has a fine, delicately sour taste, which it gets from special lactic acid bacteria. The special feature of these lactic acid bacteria is that they only allow part of the milk to curdle. The protein whey remains dissolved and is enclosed by the solid substances of the milk. This gives the yoghurt its typical, fresh taste.

Kimchi

Kimchi is a benefit for our intestinal flora. Numerous microorganisms live in it. The Korean pickled cabbage strengthens the good bacteria and stimulates digestion. The basic ingredient in most recipes is Chinese cabbage, sometimes radish. The other ingredients may vary. These include mushrooms, leek, bean sprouts, cucumber, ginger, shrimps, garlic or chilli.

The end product is a foodstuff which, in addition to its probiotic bacteria, contains minerals, vitamins and fibre.

Not without reason, Kimchi is one of the healthiest foods of all.

Kombucha

Kombucha is fermented tea. The way it's fermented makes it so special. Green tea, black tea or herbal tea (or ginseng). Special strains of bacteria, yeast fungi or the Kombucha fungus are added, which in combination with some sugar start to ferment. The resulting bioactive substances give the Kombucha its health-promoting effect. During fermentation, a gelatinous "tea fungus" called yeast or scoby forms on the surface of the preparation liquid. The acetic acid produced during fermentation and the polyphenols it contains give Kombucha an antibacterial effect. Kombucha is healthy because a large number of secondary plant substances have an antioxidant effect in the body. Antioxidants break down free radicals, prevent cell damage and can probably even have a positive effect on liver toxicity.

3.10 Nutritional components

3.10.1 Water

High quality water is the beginning and basis of everything. People no longer trust the quality from the tap—and rightly so. The increasing sales of water filters prove this. Many waterworks in this country claim that water from the tap can be drunk without hesitation. The limits for harmful substances are being raised almost every year.

It is a fact that drinking water contains high concentrations of pollutants such as heavy metals, pesticides, hormones, drug residues and recently, even sweeteners. Our body needs high-quality drinking water in large quantities in order to serve as a basic substance for maintaining vital functions. Pure, living water is increasingly becoming a scarce commodity. Therefore, it is important to make sure that it is obtained from deep springs if possible.

Still, mineral water, which is filled in plastic bottles, tend to be contaminated. Recent studies have found pathogens for meninges, urinary tract and lung diseases in them. Two thirds of all types of water sold are filled in PET bottles.

Chemicals in plastics have hormone-like effects on humans. The choice of water type directly influences the success or failure of your health efforts. Other functions of water: It keeps the blood fluid, serves as a coolant and is instrumental in detoxification. The recommended daily drinking quantity is 4% of body weight.

3.10.2 Carbohydrates
3.10.2.1 good | bad carbohydrates

Good carbohydrates and bad carbohydrates: Of course it is not quite that simple. There are big differences when it comes to carbohydrates. It is divided into simple and complex carbohydrates. For example, if we eat a slice of bread or potatoes, a lot of insulin is released to transport the carbohydrates into the cells. Insulin, however, is responsible for the storage of abdominal fat and inhibits the burning of fat, making it more difficult to burn fat. It is important to eat foods rich in carbohydrates that do not cause the blood sugar level to skyrocket. Eating a slice of wholemeal bread with cheese has less effect on your blood sugar level than eating a slice of white bread with jam. Wholemeal products contain more fibre, which makes you feel fuller for longer and ensures a healthy digestion. Pulses, vegetables and cereals are rich in fibre.

Not completely forbidden—food that you should still restrict strongly:

White bread
Noodles from white flour
Potatoes
Sweets
Cakes & Biscuits
Fast food
Chips
Alcohol
Juice & Lemonades

Carbohydrate-rich foods that you should access regularly:
Oatmeal
Wholemeal pasta
Wholemeal bread
All vegetables, few potatoes
Millet
Quinoa
Nuts

3.10.2.2 Sugar | Economic factor and production

Sugar production is an important economic factor. 30,000 farms live from sugar beet cultivation. From October to December, harvesters pull sugar beets out of the ground. 180,000 people live from sugar production. Turnover is estimated at 20 billion euros. Corresponding lobby work is being done.

The Sugar Association systematically disseminates misinformation on calorie consumption, nutritional behaviour and the health consequences instead of sticking to the facts. The importance of a balanced diet is deliberately played down.

Production:

For the production of white sugar, the cleaned and crushed sugar beets are placed in high towers in contact with plenty of hot water. Milk of lime clarifies the juice, and small particles as well as floating particles can be removed. This juice contains 16%-21% sucrose. Water is then removed from the beet juice to thicken it. At this moment, the so-called seed crystals are added to the mixture to allow the sugar to crystallise. Centrifugation produces white sugar crystals. This process is repeated several times until white household sugar is produced, consisting of 1:1 fructose glucose. 1/8 of the sugar production goes to supermarkets. The rest goes to the industry and ends up in a long list of jelly babies, chocolate, sausage, canned food and finished products.

3.10.2.3 What sugar triggers in the body

Sugar can contribute to the development of type 2 diabetes. Normal household sugar consists of glucose and fructose. When we eat it, it is broken down. Dextrose does not take long to enter the bloodstream. The pancreas then produces the hormone insulin. This hormone acts like a door opener for fructose. It is burned in the cells and energy is produced. If we constantly consume too much sugar, a kind of congestion occurs. A lot of insulin is produced, but hardly any sugar is used. Like a broken lock, the cells no longer open and close reliably over time. If the sugar remains permanently in the blood, organs and vessels are damaged.

3.10.2.4 Unmasking sugar traps | Changing shopping

When you visit the supermarket, try to buy products that are as fresh as possible and appropriate to the season. Sugar serves as a cheap filler and flavor enhancer. That is why almost all ready meals contain a lot of it. As a reminder, the maximum amount of sugar recommended by the World Health Organization is 25g per day.

3.10.2.5 hidden sugar in food

The term sugar does not always appear as such in the list of ingredients, but can hide behind many terms. In addition to ingredients that have "sugar" in their name, food manufacturers also use other types of sugar or sweetening elements, some of which are difficult to recognise as sugar because of their complicated-sounding chemical names.

3.10.2.6 Sugar alternatives
3.10.2.6.1 Honey

Honey is not far from crystal sugar. Nevertheless honey has slight advantages. It has an antibacterial effect and especially, the somewhat darker varieties contain plenty of antioxidants that counteract free radicals. Interesting for allergy sufferers: By consuming local honey, one takes in pollen from the environment all year round. Thus in many cases the irritation and reaction during the blossoming period is minimized.

3.10.2.6.2 Brown sugar

Brown sugar is the same as white sugar. The only difference is that a last step of purification was omitted. Some brown syrup still sticks to the sugar crystals. Healthwise there are neither advantages nor disadvantages, the calorie content is comparable. The only difference is that it tastes slightly like caramel and malt.

3.10.2.6.3 Agave syrup

Agave syrup is similar in structure to honey and is extracted from the Mexican agave plant. It consists mainly of fructose. Possible side effects with high consumption are flatulence and diarrhoea. Agave syrup has a high proportion of fructose, the effects of which are known (see metabolic syndrome).

3.10.2.6.4 Coconut blossom sugar

The juice of the coconut palm is used to produce sugar in the greater Asia region. It is suitable for cooking, baking and can be used in drinks. Its calorific value is comparable to that of our white household sugar. The effect on the blood sugar level is similar. It contains traces of vitamins and minerals.

3.10.2.6.5 Date Syrup

Date syrup consists of dates, water and some lemon juice. Dates not only taste good, but are also very healthy, because dates contain not only carbohydrates and calories in the form of sugar, but also plenty of nutrients. One advantage of sweeteners that many people find interesting is that they have far fewer calories than regular household sugar. On average there are up to 280 calories per 100g of date syrup. By comparison, 100g of sugar contains around 400 calories. The syrup also provides other nutrients that household sugar lacks. Among these are about 1.2g protein and up to 1.4g dietary fibre per 100g.

3.10.2.6.6 Maple syrup

This sweet juice comes from Canada. There the sap of the maple tree is tapped. For 1l syrup you need about 40l of tree sap. The lighter the concentrate, the higher the quality. Furthermore, maple syrup has a number of secondary plant substances such as potassium, iron and magnesium. Nutritionally, it is to be classified as honey.

3.10.2.6.7 Rice syrup

Rice honey, or rice sugar, is made by boiling rice flour with water to make syrup. Its sweetening power as well as its energy content is somewhat weaker than our household sugar. Vegans use it as an alternative to honey. Since the syrup contains almost no fructose, it is suitable for people with fruit sugar intolerance.

3.10.2.6.8 Stevia

Stevia is a subtropical branch species, originally from Paraguay and has been used there for centuries. It does not cause caries and therefore does not harm the teeth. Its sweetening power is up to 300 times stronger than the crystal sugar we know. Stevia is suitable for diabetics and keeps the blood sugar level constant. If you think that Stevia is a natural product, you are mistaken. The production process is highly industrialised, using environmentally harmful aluminium salts. Care should be taken when buying Stevia, some products contain normal household sugar.

3.10.2.6.9 Birch sugar (xylitol)

The extraction of xylitol is based on the chemical modification of wood sugar. This occurs in nature, for example, in coconuts, corn cobs, straw and as a waste product in paper production.

Xylitol is used in the food industry, as a sugar substitute and, unlike ordinary household sugar, has no harmful effects on the teeth. It is similar to sugar in taste and has almost the same sweetening power. Birch sugar only metabolises little insulin and is therefore suitable for diabetics. At high intakes, xylitol has a laxative effect and is harmless in humans, but has caused severe side effects in animal experiments. In dogs it affects blood clotting and causes serious liver damage.

3.10.2.6.10 Erythritol

Erythritol is completely calorie-free and therefore suitable for diabetics. In addition, it is well tolerated and tooth-friendly. Unlike other sugar alcohols, erythritol does not cause flatulence, stomach ache or diarrhoea.

3.10.2.6.11 Sweetener

Tastes sweet and provides almost no calories. We are talking about sweetener. They belong to the group of "sweeteners" and have names like aspartame, saccharin or sucralose. Eleven sweeteners are approved in Europe. In contrast to normal household sugar, they sweeten 100 to 10,000 times as much. Pure sweeteners are available as small tablets, liquid and "scattered sweeteners". They are also found in a wide variety of foods, which often advertise with references such as "light", "diet" and "sugar-free". For example, fruit yoghurts, puddings, sweets, chewing gum, jams and fruit preservatives may contain sweeteners. They are also used in calorie-free soft drinks.

The sweeteners approved in Europe are considered harmless to health. However, recent studies indicate that sweeteners favor bad intestinal bacteria and thus damage the immune system. The European Food Safety Authority reviews all food additives before they are approved. Experts set an acceptable daily intake (ADI) for sweeteners. As a rule, the ADI values are based on results from animal experiments. The amount that animals can ingest over a long period of time without causing adverse reactions is considered the basis. For example, if an animal can easily consume one gram of sweetener per kilogram of body weight per day, this amount is divided by 100 to be on the safe side. For humans, the ADI is then 0.01 g or 10 milligrams per kilogram of body weight. Once the sweeteners have been approved, expert committees will examine them as necessary. Aspartame, for example, was suspected a few years ago of causing headaches, allergies or even cancer. The suspected connections were then examined and disproved in 2013.

The following sweeteners are currently authorised in the EU:

E 950 (acesulfame K)

E 951 (aspartame)

E 952 (cyclamate)

E 954 (saccharin)

E 955 (sucralose)

E 957 (Thaumatin)

E 959 (neohesperidine DC)

E 960 (steviol glycosides)

E 961 (neotame)

E 962 (salt of aspartame-acesulfame)

E 969 (Advantam)

Behind the theory that sweeteners help you gain weight is the idea that insulin secretion is promoted and this in turn promotes cravings. The extent to which sweeteners influence the sugar metabolism is still being investigated. Major professional societies agree: sweetener is officially safe in the recommended amounts.

For me, they are among the worst alternatives, as there are already studies on the cancer risk associated with sweeteners. Sweeteners are produced purely synthetically and have an indirect influence on the intestinal environment and thus the immune system.

3.10.3 Protein | Protein

3.10.3.1 vegetable protein reduces mortality rate

Animal and vegetable protein in our food have different effects on our health. In people with existing heart disease, the consumption of animal protein has increased the mortality rate, whereas vegetable protein has developed a protective effect. If the energy intake of the test subjects increased by ten percent through dairy products, eggs and meat, the mortality rate through cardiovascular disease increased by eight percent.

If, on the other hand, it was lowered and the proteins came from bread, pulses and pasta, the mortality rate fell. The connection between protein consumption and mortality rate, however, only applies to people who live rather unhealthily overall.

Protein is not only found in fish, meat and eggs, but also in vegetable foods such as legumes and cereal products. Proteins ensure lasting satiation, whereas carbohydrates promote a renewed feeling of hunger after a short time. This is the reason why you should fall back on vegetable protein during possible phases of weight loss. Protein is involved in the formation of bones and muscles. They are formed from amino acids, the smallest building blocks, and are made available to your body in many variations. One gram of protein per kilogram of body weight per day is recommended. This means that a person of normal weight of 80kg has a requirement of 80g of protein. For older and sick people the requirement increases by 1.5g. Different rules apply to athletes and pregnant women. In case of overweight the amount is reduced by 10%.

Protein of animal origin, e.g. parmesan, turkey breast, curd cheese or chicken egg, is more similar to body protein and therefore has a higher biological value. This means that the body can use it more easily to produce the body's own protein. However, vegetable protein is healthier because it contains fibre and secondary plant substances. People with kidney disease should be cautious about eating protein, as the protein breakdown products can put an excessive strain on the kidneys.

3.10.4 Oils | Fats

Fats in food are of varying quality and account for about 35 % of the total energy intake through food. These are divided into saturated, monounsaturated and polyunsaturated fats. In addition, they are divided into animal and vegetable fats. Worth mentioning are products that have been strongly changed by the industry, so-called trans fats. Trans fats are correctly called trans fatty acids. Hardened fats such as margarine contain trans fatty acids as a component. Chemically speaking, trans fats are unsaturated fatty acids that have a double bond between two carbon atoms. They are formed during the chemical hardening of fats, are highly inflammation-promoting and pose other dangers.

Saturated fats

serve our body primarily to supply energy, are mainly found in foods of animal origin (e.g. sausage or butter) and play a major role in fat metabolism disorders, as they increase cholesterol levels. According to the recommendations of nutritional physicians, saturated fatty acids should not exceed approx. 10 % of the daily food energy. At a reference level of 2,000 kilocalories per day, this corresponds to approximately 20 to 27 grams of saturated fatty acids.

We need monounsaturated fats for the functions of our cell membranes. They are particularly abundant in rapeseed and olive oil. Monounsaturated fatty acids have a positive influence on fat metabolism.

3.10.5 Omega 3, 6 and 9 fatty acids
3.10.5.1 Omega 3 fatty acids
They belong to the unsaturated compounds and are a subgroup within the omega fatty acids. Omega 3 fatty acids are essential and must therefore be supplied from outside. The former name is vitamin F. The highest concentrations are found in vegetable oil: Linseed oil

56-71%, chia oil up to approx. 64% and perilla oil approx. 60%. Perilla oil is obtained from the seeds of the perilla plant. The plant originates from East and Southeast Asia and is mainly cultivated in India, China, Japan and Korea. The leading fish species are salmon, anchovy, sardine and herring. Fish absorb the fatty acids EPA (eicosapentaenoic acid) and DHA (docosahexaenoic acid) through their algae diet, but can also produce them themselves. The functions of DHA include protection against inflammation and infection, a healthy metabolism and support for the immune system. Furthermore, these hormones produce and regulate blood pressure. A sufficient intake of Omega 3 fatty acids through food is hardly possible. Up to 70 percent of the population is undersupplied. In contrast, the intake of unfavorable omega 6 fatty acids is disproportionately high.

3.10.5.2 Omega 6 fatty acids

Just like omega 3 fatty acids, omega 6 fatty acids perform important tasks in the human body. They also belong to the unsaturated essential fatty acids. This kind of fatty acids lower the bad LDL-Cholesterin value, however, also the good HDL values. In addition, they are involved in the regulation of blood pressure, growth and repair processes and in the control of part of the immune defence, in the form of arachidonic acid activities. This positive property is reversed, as the intake of omega 6 fatty acids is disproportionately increased. Omega 6 fatty acids must also be supplied from outside. Due to the way we eat today, however, it is almost impossible to get into an undersupply. Meat, safflower oil, corn oil and sunflower oil are rich in omega 6 fatty acids. A lack of omega 6 fatty acids leads to anaemia, susceptibility to infections, fatty liver and impaired wound healing.

3.10.5.3 Omega 9 fatty acids

A lack of omega 9 is unlikely because the body can produce the fatty acids itself. They are therefore not essential. Omega 9 fatty acids that can be taken in with food are erucic acid, gondoic acid, ximetic acid, nervonic acid and oleic acid. Oleic acid is the most important representative of this group and is mainly found in olive oil. Terms such as omega-9 fatty acids, monounsaturated fatty acids and oleic acid are often used interchangeably.

Blood lipids include LDL, HDL and triglycerides. LDL and triglycerides store fats in the blood vessels. HDL in turn breaks down the fats. An increased concentration of triglycerides and LDL cholesterol can lead to calcification and blockage of the vessels and thus to arteriosclerotic diseases.

Oleic acid has a positive influence on the ratio between HDL and total cholesterol, on HDL itself and on triglycerides. Fatty acid is also known as the "good cholesterol". Furthermore, omega-9 fatty acids are responsible for nerve conduction, the formation of hormones and the formation of cell membranes.

3.10.5.4 Relationship Omega 3 to Omega 6

There is an Omega 3 deficiency in our diet. Both omega-3 and omega-6 fatty acids regulate processes in the blood vessels and are involved in inflammatory processes. While omega-3 fatty acids dilate blood vessels, improve blood flow and inhibit inflammation, omega-6 fatty acids have the opposite effect. They constrict the blood vessels, promote blood clotting and have an anti-inflammatory effect.

Due to an excess of Omega 6 fatty acids in our modern food, Omega 3 to Omega 6 fatty acids are found in a ratio of 1:20 or higher. This leads to an overreaction of the immune system, permanent alert and latent inflammation. Researchers assume that our ancestors, as hunter-gatherers, had a ratio of omega 3 to omega 6 of 1:3—this is the ratio that evolution has designed our bodies for. When both fatty acids are in balance, we speak of a state that is neutral to inflammation and beneficial to health.

3.10.6 Vital substances

These can be divided into three different main groups: Vitamins, minerals or trace elements and secondary plant substances, also called bioactive substances.

3.10.6.1 Vitamins

Vitamins belong to the micronutrients and are organic compounds. They are involved in almost every vital process in your body. For example, in the building of muscles or the interaction of ligaments, tendons and muscles. They also contribute to the normal functioning of the nervous system and the energy balance. The majority of all vitamins are essential. This means that the body cannot produce these substances itself in sufficient quantities. That is why all essential vitamins must be taken in through food.

3.10.6.2 Minerals | Trace elements

Whether in metabolism, growth or blood formation, in the interaction of nerves and muscles—nothing works without minerals. For example, sodium and potassium regulate the water balance of our body. Calcium ensures strong bones and teeth. Iron is important for blood formation. And iodine maintains the function of the thyroid gland.

It is important that we are sufficiently supplied with all minerals, because one mineral cannot replace the other. With a balanced, varied diet in the sense of the food pyramid, this is no problem.

3.10.6.3 secondary phytochemicals

Secondary plant substances are found exclusively in plant foods. Although they are not essential for life, they mostly have health-promoting effects and are also known under the umbrella term "health-promoting substances". Secondary plant substances partly have very similar properties to vitamins.

So far, about 30,000 different secondary plant compounds with a wide range of effects are known. Important representatives are e.g. carotenoids, glucosinolates, phytosterols and flavonoids. Secondary plant compounds are found in fruits and vegetables, legumes, (wholemeal) cereals, herbs and spices, vegetable oils, nuts, seeds, teas and coffee.

3.10.7 Flavor enhancers & Co.

Flavor enhancer

Glutamate is considered an indirect thickener. It causes disorders in appetite regulation and is therefore responsible for the risk of obesity and overweight. It stimulates growth control in the brain, at the same time inducing an artificial feeling of hunger and giving foods a meaty, spicy taste. Up to one and a half million tons of this "spice" are produced and processed annually. It is suspected of causing diseases such as Alzheimer's, dementia and multiple sclerosis. The neurotoxic effect of this substance is believed to be responsible for the death of brain cells. Glutamate is often not declared on the packaging. The food industry also hides the dangerous powder behind terms like seasoning salt or flavor enhancer.

Our brain is normally protected from the penetration of toxic substances by the blood-brain barrier. However, some substances—and glutamate in particular—can penetrate this natural protective mechanism.

Preservatives

More than 300 of these additives are permitted in the EU. Each substance has been tested and classified as "safe".

E210-213: Benzoic acid and certain salts, they are suspected to cause allergies.

E220:Sulphur dioxide, can cause allergic reactions, headaches and digestive problems.

E221-228: Sulphites are sulphur compounds which can cause nausea and allergies, as well as asthma attacks.

E339, E340, E341, E450, E451, E452: Behind this are various phosphates. They are suspected of straining the kidneys and promoting arteriosclerosis.

Dyestuffs

To give food an intense color, the industry has long been using natural substances, but also artificial ones. The latter in particular can be harmful to health.

E104: Quinoline yellow may promote ADHD in children.
E127: Erythrosine red can irritate the thyroid gland, additionally like E104 it can increase ADHD.
E180: Litholrubin red belongs to the azo dyes and can cause allergies.

4. Autoimmune disease | gout | rheumatism

4.1 Nutrition in autoimmune disease

Almost all of the 80 known autoimmune diseases lead to chronic inflammation. They occur when the body's own immune system mistakenly attacks its own central nervous system. Information is either not passed on at all or only incompletely. This leads to muscle weakness, paralysis, balance problems, coordination problems and numbness. Mood swings, tiredness, trembling are also among the complications—conventional medical diagnosis incurable. However, many autoimmune diseases can be improved by intestinal therapy. The intestinal flora is a highly complex system of microorganisms.

Once the importance of nutrition is understood, improvements in the quality of life can be achieved through targeted adjustments in lifestyle and food intake. Short chain fatty acids are formed in the intestine from dietary fibres. They are able to prevent inflammation in the body and protect against an attack on the human organism and its cells. The intestinal flora plays an extremely important role, especially due to the bacterial breakdown of plant fibres and the production of numerous metabolic products that take over various tasks in the body. Short-chain fatty acids, which include acetate, propionate and butyrate, go directly to the brain, where they are responsible for the supply and repair of nerve cells.

It is therefore important to specifically support the intestinal flora in performing its protective function. The use of probiotics can be helpful here. Probiotic bacteria are included in a number of fermented foods. The following foods all contain Lactobacillus, which belongs to the useful intestinal bacteria. They are: yogurt, kefir, kimchi, sauerkraut, kombucha or fermented tea.

4.2 Nutrition for gout

Gout is a metabolic disease caused by an increased uric acid concentration (hyperuricemia) in the blood. In most cases gout is hereditary (primary hyperuricemia). In rare cases it is the consequence of other diseases (secondary hyperuricemia). Alcohol consumption and the consumption of purine-rich foods have long been known as triggers in connection with gout attacks. Purines are important building blocks of nucleic acids besides pyrimidines. Their task is to store and exchange genetic information, the blueprint of the respective organism, and to pass it on to future generations. They are not essential, but are formed by ourselves. Food of animal origin contains many purines. They are metabolized in us to uric acid and excreted via the kidneys. In case of predisposition (hyperuricemia), the intake of uric acid should be reduced to about 500mg per day. In order not to exceed this value, it is recommended to consume 150g of meat, fish or sausage at most once a day.

It is best to avoid offal completely, as it contains the highest concentration of uric acid. Excessive alcohol consumption often causes gout attacks—for several reasons. The overacidification of the blood is promoted by the formation of lactic acid. This is followed by increased crystallisation of sodium urate, which is deposited in the joints and can be very painful. Alcohol inhibits the excretion of uric acid via the kidneys and stimulates the body's own uric acid synthesis through the increased breakdown of the so-called adenine nucleotides in the liver. Beer in combination with a high-fat diet is equally unfavorable. 170mg uric acid equivalent are contained in half a litre of this drink. Low carb, fasting or ketone gene diets lead to the formation of ketone body in the blood and inhibited excretion of uric acid. In addition to these recommendations, a balanced diet with as little purine-rich food as possible, such as seafood, offal and meat, is recommended.

4.3 Nutrition for rheumatism

Rheumatism sufferers have different nutritional needs than healthy people. The right choice of food can reduce health problems with inflammatory rheumatism and help to save on medication. Overall, care should be taken to ensure a complete diet. Diets that are too one-sided should be avoided because they cause the body to suffer from a nutrient deficiency and thus provide a target for rheumatism.

Nutrition is only one component of rheumatism therapy. First and foremost it is important to severely restrict sausage and meat products. The focus is on low-fat dairy products, fish and vegetable raw materials. Food containing arachidonic acid should be avoided, as it forms inflammation-promoting messenger substances that promote inflammation in joints. This acid is found exclusively in food of animal origin, for example in dairy products and sausages. Fish, on the other hand, is a food to be preferred, because fish oil contains eicosapentaenoic acid, a fatty acid which, according to studies, can bring about an alleviation of the disease. Swollen joints and pain were relieved by eating about 800 grams of fish per week. Walnut oil, soybean oil, wheat germ oil, rapeseed oil and linseed oil also contain eicosapentaenoic acid. A third way to reduce arachidonic acid is to include fresh herbs and spices e.g. ginger, curry, garlic, caraway, as vegetable antioxidants in the daily diet.

5. You should avoid this

5.1 Noise pollution

Unlike the eyes, the ear cannot be closed. Therefore, every sound wave and tone must be evaluated and processed by the brain. Mental illnesses, diabetes or sleeping problems are just some of the consequences of excessive noise exposure. Researchers have found that constant exposure to noise from cars, trains or planes can lead to heart disease, damage to blood vessels and silent inflammation. Changes in hormone balance and other brain wave activities have been observed. Stress hormones are released, sleep is impaired and high blood pressure and heart attacks occur as a result of this exposure.

5.2 Environmental toxins | plasticizers | plastics

Environmental toxins

Eight million people in developing and emerging countries die every year as a result of contact with contaminated air, contaminated water or contaminated soil. Toxins are just as common in this country—from air and food to furniture or drinking water. It seems impossible to completely avoid contact with toxins. However, you can sharpen your awareness to reduce the impact to a minimum. Highly dangerous pesticides are a cause of health and environmental damage worldwide, with massive consequences for the integrity of people. The most harmful environmental toxins include mercury, hexavalent chromium, radionuclides, pesticides and cadmium.

Plasticizer

Plasticizers (phthalates) are a group of industrial chemicals that give flexibility and resistance to consumer and construction products, especially those made of polyvinyl chloride (PVC) or vinyl plastic. About 90% of the plasticizers are used in vinyl and are widely used. They can leach, migrate, evaporate and accumulate in household dust. Many plasticizers influence the male sex hormone through their hormone-like effect. A disturbance of testosterone activity, especially at the beginning of life, can have irreversible effects on male reproduction. Infertility, reduced sperm count and testicular atrophy have been observed in male animals.

Plastic

Plastic food containers are full of harmful chemicals. Plastics are made from refined crude oil and contain chemicals such as BPA (Bisphenol-A), which act mainly as plasticizers to make plastic more durable and flexible. Although this makes plastic practical for everyday use, it poses a significant risk to health, especially when it comes in contact with food.

When plastic containers are used for storage or heating, chemicals from the containers can get into the food. Studies have shown that high doses of BPA cause a number of serious health problems, including diabetes, heart disease and liver damage. To (supposedly) solve this problem, companies have started to produce plastic that is labelled "BPA-free". In these products BPA is replaced by other chemicals, BPS (Bisphenol-S) and phthalates such as diethylhexyl phthalate (DEHP). In many cases, however, the health risks remain. In particular, the chemicals in BPA act in a similar way to oestrogen and can, in the long term, have a lasting effect on women's hormone balance and have a negative impact on reproduction. Research has linked BPA to breast cancer in animals, along with obesity, thyroid problems and neurological disorders in humans. Contact with high concentrations of phthalates and BPA during pregnancy causes lung problems in children, which often lead to chronic asthma later on. Increased insulin resistance and increased blood pressure can also be measured in children.

5.3 Chronic stress

Stress: a constant and ever-present aggressor that attacks every tissue, especially the walls of arteries. However, it is primarily nerve damage that affects the entire organism. The inflammations caused by it develop silently without the need for infection or germ contamination. Vascular constrictions and the associated diseases angina pectoris, stroke or heart attack are the result. The human being associates stress with escape and fight. Thousands of years old evolutionary mechanisms that have been adopted in a ration of 1:1 into modern times are effective. In order to survive these situations, the body must be provided with energy. Stress systems are activated. This begins in the brain. Neurotransmitters ensure the release of rapid energy in the form of sugar. At this point, the omens of flight and fight are set. This leads to insulin release, which in turn can lead to a renewed craving for sugar. To end this cycle, it is advisable to reduce the stress level, e.g. through meditation or exercise, and to eat food that requires as little insulin as possible for metabolism. In such a situation, exercise is usually not necessary, but doing it would reduce stress and cortisol concentration in our body.

5.4 Nicotine

Inflammatory processes in the mouth are triggered by smoking and complicate wound healing. The harmful substances contained in tobacco smoke increase the inflammatory potential by a factor of two to six, they constrict the blood vessels and thus the blood supply in the event of inflammation. Nicotine promotes the development of chronic inflammation and is therefore the precursor of many diseases, especially cancer. Tobacco is considered the chief cause of cancer and the polycyclic hydrocarbons and nitrosamines it contains are highly pro-inflammatory and carcinogenic.

5.5 Alcohol

Alcohol damages all organ systems. Persistent alcohol consumption leads to inflammation of the liver. Alcohol is often the cause of inflammation of the pancreas (pancreatitis) and stomach lining (gastritis). Even the smallest amounts of alcohol attack the mucous membrane cells in the mouth, esophagus and stomach. The probability of heart muscle disease and high blood pressure is significantly increased by alcohol.

6. What you can do?

6.1 Nutrition

The most important step for you is to switch to a healthy anti-inflammatory diet. The right food gives your immune system much that it needs to become stronger and fight inflammation effectively. In detail this looks like this:

Antioxidants: Secondary plant compounds, vitamin A, vitamin C, vitamin D and a plant-based diet emphasized alkaline nutrition are the cornerstones of an anti-inflammatory diet. Especially many herbs, vegetables, fruits and spices as well as berries or apples contribute to an anti-inflammatory diet.

Fermented food:

Fermentation is a method of preserving food known since time immemorial. The activity of microorganisms causes the pH value in food to drop, thus depriving it of the basis of life for a spoilage process. The best examples are yoghurt, sauerkraut or kimchi. For more information, see the relevant section of this book.

Mediterranean diet:

The so-called Mediterranean diet is often recommended by doctors. In 2019 it was voted the best form of nutrition. The main ingredients are fish, olive oil, nuts, salad and fresh vegetables. Fatty milk and red meat in large quantities are taboo. Details can be found in the section on healthy balanced nutrition.

Acid Bases Household:

the over-acidification of the body is often referred to as an inflammatory reaction. A diet low in bases also promotes inflammation due to a lack of oxygen in the inflamed tissue.

6.2 Sports | Exercise

Regular exercise helps to maintain weight and strengthens the locomotor system. It acts as an anti-inflammatory agent and stimulates an anti-inflammatory reaction. After moderate twenty-minute jogging, the amount of immune cells that produce the so-called tumor necrosis factor (TNF) decreases by 5%. The tumor necrosis factor (TNF) belongs to a group of messenger substances (cytokines) of the immune system. It plays an important role in the body's defence (e.g. against tumor cells) and in inflammatory reactions. In chronic inflammations such as rheumatic diseases or psoriasis, the subtype TNF-alpha is found in large quantities.

6.3 Shinrin Yoku

Shinrin Yoku comes from Japan and literally means "bathing in the forest". You don't really bathe in the forest, but you do immerse yourself in the green. You do this by leaving the pace of the day behind, consciously opening your senses and letting the healing atmosphere of the forest flow through your body and mind. Deep and powerful relaxation here and now is the result. Trees and plants seem to produce substances that activate the autonomic nervous system and thus contribute to lowering blood pressure. This gives our immune system a positive boost. The more diverse the vegetation in a forest is, the more ethereal substances are in the air. According to scientific studies, movement in nature also leads to an increase in natural killer cells that seek out and destroy cancer cells. This would even contribute to long-term protection against the development of cancer.

6.4 Intestinal sanitation

A large part of the immune system and many defence reactions originate in the intestine. Alcohol, medication, bad food and stress can cause lasting damage to the intestinal flora and cause a delicate imbalance. As a result, pathological symptoms or diseases occur. An intestinal rehabilitation is always a good idea if the intestine is to be cleansed of harmful substances. An intestinal rehabilitation is divided into three parts: First the intestine is cleaned, then toxins are removed and finally the intestinal flora is rebuilt.

Intestinal rehabilitation has its origins in natural medicine. First, the intestine is emptied in several steps, cleaned of toxins and bacteria and then rebuilt to achieve a healthy intestinal environment. Such a cure requires sufficient time. This procedure can be helpful after longer phases of taking medication, a change of diet, abdominal pain and constipation. Intestinal cleansing, on the other hand, is a quick cleansing and is usually carried out in connection with an intestinal rehabilitation. From a purely orthodox medical point of view, intestinal cleansing is not a recognized form of therapy and takes one to three months. The first improvements should already be noticeable after 14 days. An intestinal rehabilitation is divided into three steps. The first step is an extensive intestinal cleansing. In the second step, acids and free radicals are bound with the help of silicate. Zeolite and bentonite transport heavy metals and drug residues from the body. In the third and last step, probiotics are used to reestablish desired intestinal bacteria and promote their growth. Yoghurt, whey, sauerkraut, apple vinegar or kimchi, for example, support this process.

6.5 Yoga | Meditation

The health care system has been recording increases in stress-related absenteeism for a long time. Of the average 15 days of incapacity to work, slightly more than 2 days are attributable to anxiety, stress disorders and depression. Every sixth child and every 5 adolescents show pronounced signs of stress. What is the reason why more and more people are overwhelmed with their everyday life? Stress significantly shortens our life expectancy and increases the risks of a whole range of diseases caused by silent inflammations such as autoimmune diseases, depression or strokes. It is always a question of the individual dose, which amount of stress is still healthy for a particular person.

6.6 Sleep

Too much or too little sleep is associated with a whole range of health problems. Research also shows that inflammation can be triggered. Sleeping at the wrong time or not enough sleep leads to numerous health problems. Too much sleep also seems to promote inflammatory activity. It is often difficult to determine what causes inflammation. However, sleep and sleep rhythm seem to play a central role. Essential repairs take place in the body during sleep. Toxins and metabolic residues are removed. Hormones associated with our sleep, e.g. melatonin, interact with antioxidants. Due to the insufficient repair of cells, they are damaged over time, leading to an increase in the inflammatory molecule cytokine. In animals, sleep deprivation also leads to the release of cytokines, which in turn leads to an immune response. There is still a belief that excess sleep is beneficial to health and would inhibit inflammation. This assumption is wrong. There is a biological reason for this. Our body reacts to too much sleep with the same release of the inflammatory molecule cytokine. For most people, seven to eight hours of sleep is the right amount.

7. Recipes

The quantities in the recipes are expressed in grams (g). Millilitre (ml) corresponds to gram (g). If this is not the case, it is mentioned separately.

7.1 Salads & Bowls

7.1.1 Chickpea salad - smoked salmon strips

You need:

500g of pre-cooked chickpeas, half a skin of cherry tomatoes, two spring onions, 100g of smoked salmon, two shallots, half a bunch of leaf parsley, 30g of olive oil, juice and skin of one lemon, salt, pepper, two red peppers, half a bunch of fresh mint.

And here we go:

Pour the chickpeas through a sieve and rinse several times. Halve the cherry tomatoes and marinate them with salt, pepper and a little sugar. Clean the spring onions and cut into fine strips. Do the same with the shallots. Wash the parsley leaves, dab dry and chop finely. Halve the peppers, remove the core and cut into fine strips. Mix everything together in a bowl. Arrange the salad and garnish with the smoked salmon strips.

7.1.2 Corn salad - feta cheese

You need:

A kilo of panicle tomatoes, 300g feta cheese, 200g canned corn, 100g Kenya beans, two medium sized onions, 30g paprika powder noble sweet, a clove of garlic, 30g olive oil, salt, pepper.

And here we go:

Wash the tomatoes, remove the stalk and cut into large pieces. Pour the corn and Kenya beans through a sieve and wash several times with lukewarm water. Cut the cheese into large pieces. Peel the onions and cut them into fine strips. Peel and finely chop the garlic. Mix everything together in a bowl and season to taste with paprika powder, olive oil, salt and pepper. Feta cheese is a brine cheese that was originally made from sheep or goat cheese. It gets its spicy taste from maturing in a brine.

7.1.3 Spanish potato salad - olives - thyme

You need:

A kilo of potatoes cooked firm, three cloves of garlic, two shallots, 20g of olive oil, salt, pepper, half a bunch of fresh thyme, 40g of dried tomatoes, half a bunch of parsley leaves, 40g of green olives without stone.

And here we go:

Peel the potatoes and cut into cubes of about 3cm. Boil the potatoes in salted water until they are not soft but firm to the bite. Soak the dried tomatoes in some water for half an hour. Then drain the potatoes and fry them in some olive oil until golden brown, season lightly with salt.

Peel the garlic and cut into fine cubes. Peel the shallots and cut into fine strips. Wash and finely chop the parsley. Pluck the thyme. Drain the olives and cut into strips. Mix everything together in a bowl and season with salt and pepper. The essential oil of thyme, called thymol, inhibits the growth of bacteria and viruses and is therefore one of the most important remedies for coughs, colds and bronchitis.

7.1.4 Asparagus ham salad with couscous
You need:
200g white asparagus, 200g green asparagus, 100g couscous, 50g baby spinach, 30g olive oil, salt, pepper, sugar, 30g white wine vinegar. 100g Parma ham.
And here we go:
Peel the white asparagus and cut it into pieces about 3cm long. Cut the end of the green asparagus about 2cm long. Young green asparagus does not need to be peeled. Lightly roast the asparagus together in a pan, add a little water and season with salt, pepper and sugar. When still warm, mix with the vinegar. Cook the couscous according to instructions. Wash baby spinach and dry it with a kitchen towel. Mix all ingredients, season with salt and pepper and garnish with Parma ham.

7.1.5 Bulgur salad with feta and beetroot
You need:

110g bulgur, 20g dill, 10g parsley, 30g cherry tomatoes, 110g yoghurt, two eggs, 40g feta, 30g whole hazelnuts, 140g boiled beetroot, lemon, garlic, olive oil, salt, pepper.

And here we go:

Pour the same amount of hot water over the Bulgur. Salt lightly and let it swell for 15 minutes. Stir occasionally. Wash and chop the dill and parsley. Boil the eggs hard for 13 minutes. Then peel and roughly dice them. Dice the feta cheese. Roast the hazelnut kernels without fat in a hot pan. Then roughly cut into pieces. Cut the beetroot into cubes of about 3cm. Clean the garlic and cut into cubes. Season everything with salt, pepper, olive oil and garlic. Carefully mix all ingredients and put them into a suitable container, for example into preserving jars. Beetroot contains betaine and the B-vitamin folate, which together lower the cholesterol level in the blood. The effect of the tuber can prevent arterial diseases and heart disease.

7.1.6 Panzanella (Italian bread salad)

You need:

A stick of Chiabatta bread, preferably from the previous day, 500g of panicles of tomatoes, three shallots, two cloves of garlic, 30g of sugar, 30g of olive oil, salt, pepper, a fresh pot of green basil, white wine vinegar.

And here we go:

Coarsely dice the chiabatta bread and toast it in a pan with olive oil. Wash the tomatoes, remove the stalk and cut into slices. Pluck the basil roughly. Clean and slice the shallots and garlic. Mix all ingredients in a bowl and season with a little olive oil and white wine vinegar as well as salt and pepper.

7.1.7 Radish potato salad

You need:

600g waxy potatoes, 1 bunch of radishes, 4 shallots, 1 bunch of chives, 200ml vegetable stock. 1 teaspoon mustard, 60ml apple vinegar, 20ml wheat germ oil.

And here we go:

Clean the potatoes and cook them unpeeled in salted water until al dente. Peel the potatoes warm. Heat vegetable stock and add mustard and vinegar. Cut the jacket potatoes into thin slices when cold. Pour the boiling vegetable stock over the potatoes and stir carefully. Wash the radishes and use a slicer to make fine slices. Add the radishes to the potatoes - refine with sprouting oil.

7.1.8 Asparagus salad - gnocchi - wild garlic pesto

You need:

450g white asparagus, 390g gnocchi, 100g olive oil, 50g wild garlic, 20g parsley, 110g young leaf spinach, two teaspoons honey, two tablespoons pine nuts, 40g grated Parmesan cheese, salt, pepper, 30g white wine vinegar

And here we go:

Peel the asparagus and cook in salt and sugar water until al dente. Then take them out and let them cool down. Wash the spinach thoroughly. Cut the asparagus into 8cm long pieces. Fry them together with the gnocchi in a pan. Wash the parsley and wild garlic. Roast the pine nuts without fat in a pan. Make a presto with the honey, the pine nuts, parmesan, salt and pepper in a mixer. Mix the asparagus together with the gnocchi and spinach in a bowl with the vinegar and arrange on a plate.

Asparagus contains vitamin C, vitamin E and the B vitamins which are important for the nervous system. Asparagus contains asparagine acid as a special ingredient. It stimulates kidney function and thus has a draining effect. If you suffer from dropsy or overweight, it is advisable to eat asparagus.

7.1.9 Orange bread salad - chicken breast fillets

You need:

Two medium-sized shallots, half a bunch of leaf parsley, 30g agave syrup, salt, pepper, 30g olive oil, half a stick of baguette bread, five medium-sized oranges, 150g chicken breast fillet.

And here we go:

Cut the baguette bread into approx. 4cm large rough cubes. Fry in a pan with olive oil. Cut the chicken breast fillets into thin strips and fry them in some oil. Season with salt and pepper and drain on a kitchen roll. Peel and fillet the oranges. Peel the shallots and cut into fine cubes. Wash the leaf parsley, dab dry and chop finely. Mix everything in a bowl.

7.2 Healthy breakfast
7.2.1 Skyr with seeds, oranges and banana

You need:

10g coconut chips, 15g cashew nuts, 15g walnut kernels, 15g almond kernels, 15g pine nuts, a banana, 2 oranges, 600g Skyr, 10g puffed amaranth.

And here we go:

Roast the seeds and coconut chips in a pan without fat and let them cool down. Mix the juice and grated orange with the Skyr. Remove the remaining orange peel and cut into slices. Spread the Skyr on peels and sprinkle the roasted seeds on top. Decorate with amaranth.

Skyr is a speciality from Iceland, which is low in fat and at the same time rich in protein and reminiscent of low-fat curd cheese. Amaranth can be described as a pseudo grain, as it is a grass species. It is extremely healthy, forms grains that contain starch but are gluten-free.

7.2.2 Spelt bread with avocado cream and graved salmon

You need:

Two fully ripe avocados, juice of half a lemon, 180g cream cheese, a bunch of spring onions, 10g chopped parsley, salt, colorful pepper from the mill, three radishes, ⅓ Cucumber, 30g sprouts—for example radish sprouts, a box of cress, four slices of spelt wholemeal bread, 200g gravlax.

And here we go:

Wash and slice the spring onions, cut the avocado in half, remove the core, remove the flesh, crush finely with a fork. Sprinkle the avocado with the juice of the lemon so that it does not discolor. Wash, clean and slice the radish and cucumber. Mix the cream cheese with the avocado and add the parsley. Season to taste with salt, pepper and the remaining lemon. Toast wholemeal bread. Spread the avocado cream on top and cover with slices of radish and cucumber. Place the salmon on top and garnish with radish sprouts and cress. Avocado is also called the butter of the forest because of its high fat content. This fruit has a high content of unsaturated fatty acids, which can be easily converted into energy by your body. While avocado also has a low fructose content.

7.2.3 Birch muesli with carrot boscope salad

You need:

25g grated coconut, 15g cashew nuts, 10g cranberries, 10g raisins, 70g oatmeal, 280g yoghurt, 20g honey, a medium boskop, a carrot, juice and grated lime, a pinch of sugar, a pinch of salt

And here we go:

Roast the cashew nuts and grated coconut in a pan without fat until golden brown. Wash the carrot and brush it under water. Wash and quarter the boskop and remove the core. Leave the skin on the apple and carrot. Cut the apple and carrot into fine strips or grate them with a suitable slicer. Marinate with sugar and salt, work through slightly and season to taste with the juice and grated lime. Mix the yoghurt, honey, oat flakes, cranberries and raisins, leave to stand for 5 minutes and fill into bowls. Decorate with Carrot boskop Salad. The boskop is a winter apple with a particularly high acid content. Those who appreciate sour apples can enjoy this apple variety fresh as table fruit. In addition, boskop apples have particularly few allergens, which is why they are edible for some apple allergy sufferers.

7.2.4 Oatmeal with maple syrup and banana

You need:

60g oat flakes, 250g oat milk, 40g maple syrup, half a teaspoon of cinnamon, one banana, 20g walnuts or pine nuts, 10g oat flakes, 10g icing sugar.

And here we go:

Bring oat milk to boiling point in a pot, add oat flakes, stir well and allow to swell for 5 minutes. Add maple syrup and cinnamon. Make sure that nothing burns. Roast the walnuts or pine nuts and the oat flakes in a pan without fat. Caramelize with icing sugar. Spread the oatmeal porridge on peels and decorate with sliced banana and the roasted seeds. In contrast to conventional sugar, maple syrup contains some valuable minerals such as calcium, potassium, magnesium and iron. However, the energy content is only slightly lower than that of sugar and honey.

7.3 Alkaline nutrition
7.3.1 Wild herb soup

You need:

300g wild herbs (e.g. dandelion, wild garlic, sorrel), 120g leek, 80g celery, 100g carrots, 2 shallots, salt, pepper, 100 ml cream, 80g butter, 40g wholemeal spelt flour

And here we go:

Wash and clean the vegetables and cut into large cubes. Wash wild herbs and dry with a kitchen towel. Heat 40g butter in a pot and sauté the cleaned vegetables in it. Add 500ml water and the cream. Season with salt and pepper. Knead remaining butter with the wholemeal spelt flour. Cook the vegetables for about 15 minutes and puree them with a hand blender. Add the flour butter and seduce with a whisk. Cook for another 5 minutes. Separate the wild herbs finely. Keep a small part for decoration. Add the remaining part to the soup and puree with a hand blender. Serve on plates and decorate with the remaining wild herbs.

7.3.2 Grilled vegetables with rocket salad

You need:

190g of mushrooms, 210g of carrots, 220g of courgettes, 1800g of aubergines, 200g of pickled artichokes, 200g of shallots, 450g of dark Aceto Balsamico, 180g of sugar, salt, pepper, three cloves of garlic, 140g of olive oil, 310g of rocket, 200g of Parma ham, sliced.

And here we go:

Wash and clean the vegetables and cut them into sticks. Cut large mushrooms in half. Fry the vegetables one after the other in olive oil, season with sugar, add vinegar and vegetable stock. Let the vegetables cool down, store them separately and season with salt, pepper and garlic. Place grilled vegetables alternately with rocket and Parma ham in large glasses or suitable containers.

7.3.3 Melon Granite

You need:

1/4 watermelon, juice and peel of two limes, 30g agave juice.

And here we go:

Clean the watermelon and put only the pure pulp in the container of a blender. Wash the limes, grate the peel. Finely puree them all together with the agave syrup and freeze them on a flat baking tray. From time to time, use a spatula to remove the frozen ice from the tray until an ice cream mass is formed.

7.3.4 Oven vegetables

You need:

300g aubergine, 300g courgettes, 300g brown mushrooms, 300 g yellow and red peppers, 3 red onions, 4 cloves of garlic, 50g olive oil, rock salt, pepper, 3 sprigs of rosemary.

And here we go:

Wash and clean all vegetables. Cut the aubergine and zucchini into 2cm thick slices. Cut the bell peppers into thick strips, peel the red onion and quarter it. Do not wash the mushrooms, just clean them. Mushrooms behave like sponges and lose a lot of their taste and consistency when washed. Mix all vegetables in a large bowl with salt, pepper, olive oil, garlic and the rosemary very well and cook on a baking tray at 180 degrees for about 40 minutes.

7.4 Soups

7.4.1 Pumpkin turnips soup

You need:

360g pumpkin, 300g turnips, an onion, a clove of garlic, a red pepper, a bunch of spring leek, 800g vegetable stock, 40g rapeseed oil, 10g paprika powder, 10g curry powder, 10g chili powder, salt, sugar, pepper, 40g white wine vinegar.

And here we go:

Wash the pumpkin, remove the skin and cut into pieces of about 2cm. Do the same with the turnips. Clean and chop the onions and bell pepper. Heat the pumpkin, turnips and onion in a medium pot together with the rapeseed oil and sauté the vegetables until they have taken on some color. Fill up with the vegetable stock. Let the soup cook for about 20 minutes. Flavor with salt, sugar, pepper, white wine vinegar, powder and paprika powder to taste slightly sweet and spicy.

Pumpkin shows its effect in cardiovascular diseases and high blood pressure; carotenoids and dietary fibres reduce the risk of cardiovascular diseases. The potassium content strengthens the heart, as it protects it against high blood pressure.

7.4.2 Beetroot sweet potato soup

You need:

130g sweet potatoes, 200g beetroot, pre-cooked, 130g waxy potatoes, one medium onion, 20g butter, one orange, 30g ginger, 10g garlic, 1l water, curry powder, coriander, paprika powder, turmeric, 100g chickpeas pre-cooked, 150g cream, one litre vegetable stock.

And here we go:

Peel the sweet potatoes and cut into cubes of about 1cm. Drain the beetroot and cut into cubes. Peel and dice the potatoes. Clean and chop the onion. Grate orange peel and press orange. Clean ginger and garlic and chop finely. Sweat sweet potatoes, potatoes, onions, ginger, garlic in some butter. Fill up with vegetable stock. Add chick peas. Puree with a blender for about 5 seconds. Add the cream. Bring to the boil and season to taste with curry powder, coriander, paprika powder, turmeric, salt and pepper.

7.4.3 Thais coconut soup with rice noodles

You need:

100g shiitake mushrooms, 100g baby spinach, two tablespoons lime juice, two teaspoons lime zest, two spring onions, two medium-sized carrots, 500g coconut milk, a bunch of fresh coriander, 210g rice ribbon noodles, 45g curry paste red, kaffir lime leaf, 20g rapeseed oil, salt, pepper, 100 g peanuts.

And here we go:

Clean the mushrooms and cut them into fine strips. Brush the carrot under water and peel into fine strips with a peeler. Wash the coriander and pluck finely. Grate the lime, then halve and juice it. Heat the oil and fry the curry paste lightly for 1 minute. Add milk and 450g water and bring to the boil briefly. Add the pasta. Add spring onions, carrot strips, mushrooms, kaffir lime leaf, lime juice and lime zest and cook for 5-6 minutes. Remove the kaffir leaf and add the spinach. Bring to the boil once briefly and then serve the soup immediately. Decorate with chopped peanuts and coriander. Kaffir limes are cultivated exclusively as a spice and medicinal plant and have an intense lemon flavor. The leaves are said to have antioxidant, antibacterial and anti-inflammatory properties.

7.4.4 Apple horseradish soup

You need:

Four large boskop apples, a fresh horseradish, 30g butter, 200g white wine, 400g vegetable stock, 100g cream, salt, pepper, lemon juice, a medium-sized shallot, 30g rapeseed oil, a small medium hot chilli, a small bunch of chervil.

And here we go:

Do not peel apples, cut them into quarters, remove the core and cut one apple into cubes and put it aside. Peel the horseradish using a peeler, then grate it with a kitchen grater. Sauté the apple cubes in butter and season with a little sugar. Clean the shallot and cut into cubes. Do the same with the chilli pepper. Heat rapeseed oil, fry shallots and apple cubes for 1 minute. Wash the chervil, pluck and put aside. Fill up with vegetable stock, white wine and cream. Bring to the boil and let it simmer for 5 minutes. With the help of a puree stick, thicken the soup with salt, pepper and lemon juice to taste. Finally, stir in the grated horseradish and bring to the boil briefly. Serve the soup immediately when it's still hot. Dice the caramelized apple and decorate with the chopped chervil.

7.4.5 Curry lentil soup with baked cauliflower

You need:

1l vegetable stock, 450g coconut milk, three and a half red peppers, 180g pink lentils, three medium carrots, one onion, four teaspoons of red curry paste, half a head of cauliflower, 40g olive oil, 30g curry powder, salt, pepper, 30g lemon juice.

And here we go:

Divide the cauliflower into florets and marinate with olive oil and salt. Place in the oven on a baking tray and roast at 220° C for about 20-25 minutes. Then take out and drain on a kitchen towel. Wash the peppers and cut them into cubes. Peel carrots and also cut into small cubes. Clean onion and cut into cubes. Heat the olive oil and fry the pink lentils as well as the diced onion and curry paste for about 1 minute. Fill up with coconut milk and vegetable stock. Cook for about 15 minutes at low heat. Stir again and again to prevent burning. After about 15 minutes cooking time add the carrot and the diced peppers. Season to taste with curry powder, salt, pepper and lemon juice. Serve soup hot and decorate with the baked cauliflower florets.

7.4.6 Potato mushroom soup

You need:

210g waxy potatoes, 260g mushrooms, a stick of leek (approx. 200g), 700g vegetable stock, 100g cream, a tablespoon of rapeseed oil, salt, pepper, marjoram.

And here we go:

Peel potatoes and cut into cubes. Clean and slice the mushrooms. Wash the leeks under running water until there is no sand left. Then cut into 2cm thick slices. Pluck the marjoram. Fry half of the mushrooms in some rape oil and season with salt and pepper. Dry them on a kitchen roll and put them aside for decoration. Heat the rapeseed oil in a pot, add the potatoes, mushrooms and leek and fry for about 2 minutes. Fill up with vegetable stock and cream and let it simmer for about 15 minutes at a mild heat. Use a blender to blend the soup to a creamy consistency. Season to taste with salt and pepper. Serve the soup very hot and decorate with the mushroom slices and plucked marjoram.

7.4.7 Chorizo stew

You need:

380g vine of tomatoes, 200g chorizo, four cloves of garlic, 150g potatoes, one red pepper, one green pepper, one medium zucchini, one bunch of soup greens, one spring onion, three tablespoons of tomato paste, one tablespoon of white wine vinegar, one bunch of fresh oregano, 750g vegetable stock, 30g rapeseed oil, salt, pepper.

And here we go:

Cut the chorizo into strips. Clean and wash all the vegetables and cut them into cubes of about 2cm. Heat rapeseed oil and sauté the vegetables for about 2-3 minutes. Add tomato paste and after about another minute add vegetable stock. Cook for 25-30 minutes. Season to taste with salt, pepper and chilli powder and serve hot. Be careful with the salt first because the sausage is salty. Chorizo so is a spicy, firm, coarse-grained raw sausage from Spain and Portugal based on pork, seasoned with paprika and garlic.

7.4.8 French onion soup

You need:

5 large vegetable onions, 30g butter, 20g flour, 100g white wine, 1.4 litres beef stock, 1 bay leaf, 4 stalks of thyme, salt, pepper, 8 slices of baguette, 70g grated Gruyere.

And here we go:

Peel onions and cut into strips. Sauté in melted butter. Add the flour and fry for 1 minute. Fill up with white wine and stock, add bay leaf and simmer for approx. 30 minutes at low heat. Remove the bay leaf, add the chopped fresh thyme and simmer for another 10 minutes. Arrange the soup in hot soup plates, cover with baguette slices and put grated cheese on the bread slices and bake at high top heat.

7.4.9 Minestrone

You need:

250g of white beans, a bunch of vegetables, 20g of parsley, 20g of thyme, 20g of laurel, 1 bunch of basil, 200g of olive oil, salt, 140g of grated parmesan, 60g of pine nuts.

1 medium broccoli, 1 celery, 200g of tomatoes, 40g of olive oil, 20g of tomato paste, salt, pepper, 1 small chilli pepper, 200g of green beans, 2 small carrots, 1 fennel bulb, 1 medium courgette.

And here we go:

Soak the beans overnight. On the other day, rinse and cook with the vegetable bundle, some laurel, thyme and parsley for about 2-3 hours. Do not salt, otherwise the beans will not soften. Roast the pine nuts in a pan without fat. Mix olive oil, parmesan, pine nuts in a mixer to make a pesto.

Clean the broccoli and cut into florets. Wash the celery and cut into strips. Clean and halve the beans. Peel and chop the carrots. Wash and chop the zucchini.

Sauté the vegetables in some olive oil. Add tomato paste. Add the bean stock and cook for 35 minutes. Season to taste with salt, pepper and some garlic. Serve hot together with the pesto.

7.4.10 Lentil soup with spinach

You need:

90g onions, 180g carrots, 80g celeriac, a stick of leek, 80g dates without stones, a bunch of leaf parsley, 40g olive oil, 240g mountain lentils, 1l chicken stock, a teaspoon of cinnamon, 200g baby leaf spinach, 140g yoghurt, 20g lemon juice, salt, pepper, six sticks of mint, 10g Ducca (North African spice mix), one salted lemon.

Salt lemons are a speciality of North African cuisine. The lemons are pickled in brine and are an ingredient of many traditional dishes. For the spice mixture Ducca, sesame and nuts are combined with coriander, cumin, mint and thyme.

And here we go:

Wash or clean the celery, carrots, onions and leeks and cut them into pieces about 1cm in size. Cut dates finely. Drain and thinly slice the lemon and chop finely. Wash and dry parsley and chop finely. Heat the oil in a large pot. Steam onions, carrots, celery, leek and 20g Ducca at medium heat for about 2-3 minutes. Add lentils, salt, lemon and dates. Fill up with the stock and 300g water and boil. Add cinnamon and parsley and cook over medium heat for about 50 minutes, stirring continuously. Wash the spinach and spin dry. Puree the soup lightly with a blender for about 5 seconds. Season to taste with salt and pepper, add the spinach and serve hot. Sprinkle with the yoghurt.

7.4.11 Carrot soup with spelt croutons

You need:

400g of carrots, two medium-sized onions, 100g of white balsamic vinegar, 30g of ginger, 20g of olive oil, 500g of vegetable stock, 300g of coconut milk, salt, sugar, ground white pepper, two medium-sized red chillies, two slices of spelt bread, 20g of butter, half a bunch of chives.

And here we go:

Peel carrots, peel onions and cut into cubes. Clean ginger and cut into fine strips. Cut carrots into cubes. Halve and roughly chop the chillies. Heat the olive oil in a medium pot and fry the carrots together with the ginger, onions and chillies. Fill up with the vegetable stock. Cook for about 20 minutes and then add the coconut milk and vinegar. Finish the soup with a blender. Season to taste with salt, sugar, ground pepper and chilli.

Cut spelt bread into cubes and lightly toast in butter. Serve the soup with the spelt croutons and chopped chives.

7.4.12 Parsley root soup

You need:

One kilo of parsley root, 120g floury potatoes, two medium sized onions, 40g rape seed oil, 200g dry white wine, 20g vegetable stock (instant), one medium sized apple for example boskop, 200g whipped cream, salt, pepper, nutmeg, sugar.

And here we go:

Peel and wash the parsley root and separate about 150g of it. Cut the rest roughly. Peel, wash and chop the potatoes. Peel and chop the onions. Fry the onions together with the parsley roots in a pot with hot oil. Deglaze with white wine, a quarter litre of water and the vegetable stock, then bring to the boil. After about 20 minutes add the cream and puree. Season to taste with salt, pepper, nutmeg and sugar. Fry the remaining parsley roots with the finely diced potatoes in a pan, sprinkle with a little sugar. Serve the soup and garnish with the caramelized potato and apple cubes.

7.4.13 Turnips Potato soup with wild garlic Pesto

You need:

One medium onion, 20g of rapeseed oil, 400g of rutabaga, 350g of potatoes, floury cooking, 20g of vegetable stock (instant), 20g of red curry paste, 50g of cream, 80g of pine nuts, 60g of wild garlic, 40g of olive oil, 40g of sliced Parmesan cheese, salt, pepper, sugar.

And here we go:

Wash the turnips and cut into large cubes. Do the same with the potatoes. Peel and dice the onions. Heat the rapeseed oil in a medium pot and fry the turnips together with the potatoes. Deglaze with 700g water and the vegetable stock. Add the cream and the curry paste. Use a blender to make a homogeneous soup. Lightly roast the pine nuts without fat in a pan - let them cool down. Puree together with the olive oil, wild garlic, parmesan, salt, pepper and a little sugar to a pesto. Serve the soup and garnish with pine and wild garlic pesto.

Bear's garlic is a relative of garlic, onion and chives. It has white flowers and was already known to the Romans and Germanic tribes as a spice and medicinal plant. Bear's garlic contains vitamin C, essential oils, magnesium and iron. Although it tastes similar to garlic, it does not affect mouth and body odour.

7.4.14 Lentil soup with chard and minced meat

You need:

Two medium sized peppers, a lemon, 70g of chard, 260g of pink lentils, 150g of minced beef, 20g of caraway seeds, 10g of cumin, 20g of butter, 25g of vegetable stock (instant) 10g of ginger, a clove of garlic, a medium sized onion.

And here we go:

Wash the chard, then cut into 3cm pieces. Halve the pepperoni and process into fine slices. Clean and chop the garlic clove. Remove ginger from the skin and cut into cubes. Heat butter in a medium sized pot and fry onions, garlic, ginger, cumin, caraway seeds for about 20 seconds. Add minced beef and fry gently. Add lentils, pour in water and vegetable stock. Cook over a mild heat for about 20 minutes until the mixture is smooth. Add the chard 5 minutes before the end of the cooking time. Season to taste with lemon juice, salt and pepper. Serve the soup and garnish with the pepperoni.

7.4.15 Kohlrabi Savoy Soup

You need:

200g kohlrabi, 200 g savoy cabbage, one medium onion, one medium potato, 20g butter, 100g white wine, 20g vegetable stock (instant), 100g cream cheese, salt, pepper, nutmeg, half bunch of chervil.

And here we go:

Wash, clean and dice the kohlrabi. Do the same with savoy cabbage and potatoes. Peel and chop the onion. Heat the butter in a medium pot and fry the kohlrabi, savoy cabbage, onions and potatoes. After 2 minutes, add 750g water and the white wine and vegetable stock. Season the cream cheese with salt, pepper and nutmeg and form into cams with the help of a teaspoon.

Serve the soup and garnish with the cream cheese curls and sliced chervil.

7.4.16 spicy noodle soup with chicken

You need:

Coriander seeds, one chilli pepper, dried, ¼ bunch of mint, salt, pepper, 1 onion, one green pepper green, 320g chicken breast fillet, 50g olive oil, 200g vermicelli, 2 tablespoons sugar, 350g tomatoes peeled, two leaves of bay leaf, 1 tsp. paprika powder, 1 tbsp. cumin seed, 1 tbsp. oregano, ½ tsp. ground pigment, 1.3l poultry stock, one red onion, one bunch of coriander green, one firm avocado, juice of half a lime.

And here we go:

Roast the dried chilli, cumin and coriander seeds without fat in a pan. Crush everything together with salt. Dice onion and garlic. Cut pepper without seeds into strips. Cut chicken meat into cubes of approx. 3cm and season.

Sauté the meat in hot olive oil. Add onions and garlic and fry until transparent. Add remaining spices and tomatoes to the meat. Steam for about 4 minutes until the tomatoes burst open. Add pasta and chicken stock and cook for about 20 minutes.

Cut red onions into rings. Chop the coriander. Pluck mint. Clean the avocado and cut the flesh into approx. 3cm pieces. Mix the soup with salt, pepper, coriander green, mint, diced avocado and onions and serve.

7.5 Keto Recipes

7.5.1 Fried cod on zucchini vegetables

You need:

400g of cod fillet, salt, pepper, juice of half a lemon, 400g of courgette vegetables, a vine tomato, 10g of red curry paste, 20g of olive oil.

And here we go:

Clean and wash the zucchini and then cut them into sticks of about 5-7cm length. Drain the cod on a kitchen towel and season with salt, pepper and the juice of the lemon. Wash the vine tomato, remove the greenery and cut into fine cubes. Sauté the cod in olive oil and cook in an oven at 120°. Roast zucchini vegetables in olive oil, add diced tomatoes, season with salt, pepper and the red curry paste. Arrange the zucchini tomato sticks on plates and place the cod on top.

7.5.2 Lentil roasts

You need:

190g lentils, 110g onions, 100g leeks, 100g carrots, 100g mushrooms, four tablespoons coconut flour, a teaspoon curry, salt, pepper, 40g olive oil, a small red medium hot chilli pepper.

And here we go:

Soak the lenses overnight. Clean or wash onions, carrots, leeks and mushrooms and then chop them up. Pour lentils through a sieve and drain. Clean and chop the chilli pepper. Mix all ingredients in a food processor with a fast rotating knife to a homogeneous mass.

Heat the olive oil in a pan and arrange evenly shaped lentil roasts on both sides.

7.5.3 Konjac noodles with avocadopesto

You need:

500g konjac noodles, two avocados, 100g dried tomatoes, two cloves of garlic, 90g pine nuts, half a pot of basil, 40g olive oil, salt, pepper.

And here we go:

Roast pine nuts without fat in a pan. Soak the tomatoes in lukewarm water for half an hour. Remove the flesh from the avocado. Squeeze the tomatoes. Pluck the basil. Mix all ingredients except the pasta with a hand blender to an avocado-basil pesto. Cook the cognac noodles according to instructions and fold in the avocado pesto.

Conjak noodles are especially popular in Chinese and Japanese cuisines. They are made from the kanjak root and have almost no calorific value.

7.5.4 Ketogenic almond bread

You need:

310g almond flour, 260g linseed flour, 4 eggs, 40g coconut flour, ½ cubes yeast fresh, 1 teaspoon sugar, 1 teaspoon salt.

And here we go:

Mix all ingredients and work into a homogenous dough. Cover and leave to rise in a warm place for 60 minutes. After 60 minutes, knead and leave to rise for a further 60 minutes. Preheat an oven to 180 degrees. Line a box form with baking paper and bake the dough in it for about 55 minutes. The sugar in the dough has been added to loosen it up and „feed" the yeast and is no longer present at the end of the baking process.

7.5.5 Ricotta Quiche

You need:

40g linseed flour, 10g coconut flour, 40g almond flour, 10g chia seeds, 3g psyllium husks, 80ml water, salt, 410g ricotta, a bunch of basil, a clove of garlic, three spring onions, four eggs, 100g grated Parmesan cheese, 50ml lemon juice, salt, pepper.

And here we go:

Knead psyllium husks, chia seeds, coconut flour, almond flour, linseed flour, salt and water to a dough.

Clean and slice the spring onions. Mix the ricotta together with the chopped basil, crushed garlic clove, spring onions, eggs, parmesan, lemon juice, salt and pepper. Roll out the dough and line an ovenproof dish with it. Pour in the ricotta cream and bake at 180° for 35 minutes.

7.5.6 Chicken Feta Broccoli Casserole

You need:

360g chicken breast fillet, 100g feta cheese, 200g cream, 50g pesto, salt, pepper, 150g broccoli, 30g olive oil, 120g grated Emmental cheese, 20g chopped garlic, one small red chilli pepper chopped.

And here we go:

Cut the chicken breast fillets into approx. 5cm pieces. Cut the broccoli into florets and cook in slightly salted water for about 5 minutes. Heat 20g olive oil in a pan and brown the chicken breast fillets in it. Season with salt and pepper. Dice the feta cheese.

Mix all ingredients, season with salt and pepper and bake in a casserole dish at 180° for about 45 minutes.

7.5.7 Radish spaghetti with vegetable bolognese

You need:

200g carrots, 200g courgettes, 200g celeriac, one red pepper, six shallots, two cloves of garlic, two small red medium hot chillies, 200g canned peeled tomatoes, 60g olive oil, salt, pepper, three tablespoons tomato puree, 250ml red wine, half a bunch of leaf parsley, 600g white radish.

And here we go:

Wash the carrots, celery and zucchini and cut them into fine cubes. Heat olive oil in a medium pot and fry the vegetables at medium heat for about 2-3 minutes. Add tomato paste and steam for another 2 minutes. Deglaze with red wine and boil down very strongly. Add peeled tomatoes, bring to the boil and season with salt and pepper. Cook for another 30 minutes.

Clean the radish and turn it over a spiral slicer. Heat olive oil in a suitable pan and warm the radish over a high heat. Season with salt and pepper.

Arrange the radish noodles on plates together with the vegetable bolognese.

7.5.8 Pan of vegetables with Thai asparagus

You need:

450g white asparagus, four shallots, two red peppers, 100g bamboo shoots fresh, 100g mung beans sprouts fresh, 40ml rapeseed oil, 30ml soy sauce, 30ml teriyaki sauce, 20g of ginger, two cloves of garlic, a stick of lemon grass, a small medium hot pepper, 200ml coconut milk, salt, pepper.

And here we go:

Peel the asparagus and cut into pieces of about 5cm. Clean the shallots and cut them into pieces. Halve the peppers and cut them into large pieces. Clean ginger and garlic and cut into fine pieces. Heat rapeseed oil in a frying pan. Braise asparagus, peppers, shallots, bamboo shoots, mung beans and sprouts. Add lemon grass. Deglaze with coconut milk, Teriyaki sauce and soy sauce. Reduce slightly, remove lemon grass. Arrange vegetable pan on plates.

The word „Teriyaki" is based on the Japanese words „teri" for shine and „Yku" for grilling or braising. Teriyaki sauce is mostly made from soy sauce, rice wine, honey and spices.

7.5.9 Pumpkin-Spinach-Curry

You need:

300g Butternut pumpkin, 400g fresh leaf spinach, 4 shallots, 30g fresh ginger, 2 small medium hot red chillies. 1 teaspoon cumin, 2 cloves of garlic, 30g rape seed oil, 200ml coconut milk, 200g vegetable stock, salt, pepper, juice and zest of one lemon, 10g curry powder hot.

And here we go:

Peel the pumpkin, remove seeds and dice the flesh. Wash spinach and remove thick stalks. Peel and grate ginger. Clean garlic and chop finely. Clean the chilli pepper and cut into small cubes. Peel and chop the shallots.

Heat oil and fry pumpkin, shallots, curry powder, ginger, cumin, garlic and chili for about 1 minute. Add vegetable stock and coconut milk and cook for about 20 minutes until the pumpkin is done. Add the spinach and work through briefly until the spinach has collapsed. Add salt, pepper and lemon juice to taste.

7.6 Salad dressings

Most salad dressings in supermarket refrigerated cabinets contain a variety of ingredients, including stretch, additives and preservatives. These ingredients are unhealthy, expensive and superfluous. Making salad dressings yourself is healthier and requires little effort.

7.6.1 Vinaigrette, classic
You need:
For the classic of all salad dressings one part vinegar, lemon juice or another acid and three parts oil. The oil can be based on sunflowers, rape, sesame, olives, etc. It is important that the oil is the first pressing. For frying and cooking I prefer high quality olive oil from the first pressing in organic quality. If a taste-intensive vinegar, for example old white wine vinegar, is used, a tasteless oil should be used and vice versa.

A typical basic recipe is: 100g white wine vinegar, 400g rape seed oil, half a tablespoon of mustard, a tablespoon of sugar, salt, pepper, half a teaspoon of garlic.
And here we go:
The most common mistake made when making a vinaigrette: all the ingredients are mixed together in a container with a hand blender. This procedure causes the oil to settle and the salad dressing to taste oily. The

principle is as follows: An emulator is needed, such as mustard or egg yolk. First you put a tablespoon of mustard, salt, sugar or honey, pepper, a little garlic and the white wine vinegar in the container. In the second course, stir in the oil, first drop by drop, then in larger quantities. The result will be a homogeneous, round tasting salad dressing, in which the oil will not settle permanently. If you are looking for a special variant, white wine vinegar is replaced by e.g. raspberry vinegar and the addition of fresh raspberries.

7.6.2 Yoghurt dressing

You need:

For the basic version of a yoghurt dressing: 300g yoghurt, 50g white wine vinegar, 40g rapeseed oil, two teaspoons mustard, salt, pepper and sugar or honey.

And here we go:

Mix all ingredients in a bowl and with a whisk—done. If you want to make the sauce spicier, use garlic and chilli. Another variation is to add freshly cut chives and pink pepper berries to the base. If you like it more Asian, use ginger, freshly cut coriander and cayenne pepper.

7.6.3 Blueberry pumpernickel dressing

You need:

110g pumpernickel, 140g blueberries, 120g blueberry juice, 30g apple vinegar, 60g olive oil, one orange, salt, pepper, one tablespoon blueberry jam.

And here we go:

retain half of the blueberries. Chop the pumpernickel coarsely. Grate the orange peel. Juice the orange. Mix all ingredients in a blender to a homogeneous mass.

This dressing is particularly suitable in winter as a salad dressing or marinade. Pumpernickel is a speciality from Westphalia and consists of rye meal, salt and water. Pumpernickel is baked for about 24 hours and therefore caramelised. This gives the bread its own sweet note.

7.6.4 Washabi lime dressing

You need:

100g sour cream, 110g olive oil, 200g apple juice, one tablespoon wasabi paste, one lime, a small piece of ginger root, salt, pepper, sugar.

And here we go:

Clean and finely grate the ginger, wash the lime warm and grate the peel. Halve the lime and squeeze out the ginger, lime zest, lime juice, wasabi, sour cream, apple juice in a bowl. Add olive oil slowly and then quickly. Season to taste with salt, pepper and sugar. This salad dressing reminds of a horseradish dressing. It goes very well with, for example, a lamb's lettuce with croutons and bacon.

Wasabi is green, hot, comes from the land of smiles and is also called Japanese horseradish. For a long time it was known exclusively to friends of Asian cuisine. Mixed with soy sauce, it should not be missing in any sushi dish.

7.6.5 Buttermilk blackberry dressing

You need:

100g lettuce, 100g buttermilk, 150g crème fraîche, two tablespoons balsamic vinegar, two tablespoons maple syrup, 50g fresh blackberries, salt, pepper, sugar.

And here we go:

Hold back half of the blackberries. Puree the other ingredients in a bowl using a blender. Quarter the remaining blackberries and stir into the dressing. The lettuce will bind the blackberries at this point. Alternatively, iceberg, lamb's lettuce or lollo rosso could be used.

7.6.6 Cranberry and hazelnut dressing

You need:

50g sugar, 50g cranberry, four tablespoons water, 20g medium hot mustard, 50g white wine vinegar, 50g hazelnut oil, 150g rape oil.

And here we go:

Caramelise the sugar in a small pot until brown. Add the cranberries and water, cover and simmer for about 5 minutes until the caramel has dissolved. Then let the cranberries cool down and puree them with a hand blender. Mix mustard, cranberries, vinegar, salt, sugar and pepper. Slowly stir the hazelnut oil and rapeseed oil into the mixture.

Cranberries are sweet and sour tasting berries originally from North America. They have a high content of secondary plant substances and thus have a positive effect on the intestinal flora and against urinary tract infections. Their taste is reminiscent of cranberries and they are often served as compote with game dishes at Christmas time.

7.6.7 Pea and balm dressing

You need:

100g frozen peas, a bunch of lemon balm, 20g white wine, 100g vegetable stock, 200g rape seed oil, salt, pepper, sugar.

And here we go:

Blanch deep-frozen peas in lightly salted water for about 3 minutes. Let them cool down. Mix the peas, lemon balm, white wine, salt, pepper, sugar, garlic in a container and then add the vegetable stock and finally the rape seed oil using a hand blender.

This salad dressing is perfect with rustic pasta salads, for example an Italian pasta salad with olives, cucumber, bresaola and shaved parmesan. Lemon balm is a must for any garden planting. It belongs to the classic kitchen and medicinal herbs. Its lemon fragrance makes it a popular and versatile component of traditional dishes. Its ingredients help against restlessness and stomach ailments.

7.6.8 Mango-Jalapeño Dressing

You need:

One large mango, two fresh red jalapeño, a clove of garlic, a lime, 40g of olive oil, a large red onion, 100g of orange juice, 20g of liquid honey, salt, pepper.

And here we go:

Halve the mango, remove the core, remove the mango flesh and dice coarsely. Peel and cut the garlic clove. Grate the lime peel and juice it. Peel red onion and cut into fine cubes. Wash the jalapeño, cut it in half, remove the seeds and cut into rings. Sauté the mango cubes and finely chopped jalapeño in some olive oil, add the honey. Add the juice of orange and lime as well as their abrasions. Leave to cool, then puree. Stir in olive oil and finally add red onion and the rest of the jalapeño.

Excellent with a colorful leaf salad with fried chicken breast and baguette bread. Jalapeño is one of the most popular types of chili. They are characterized by a strong but tolerable pungency. The vitamin-rich Mexican pod is often used in salsa, baked or pickled in vinegar.

7.7 Raw food

7.7.1 Gazpacho-cold tomato soup

You need:

A kilo of vine of tomatoes, half a stick of celery, a cucumber, three slices of toast, a clove of garlic, a red pepper, three tablespoons of red wine vinegar, two medium shallots, olive oil, salt, sugar, half a pot of basil, pepper.

And here we go:

Remove the crust from the bread and soak in cold water. Wash the tomatoes, remove the greenery and cut into large cubes. Wash and finely dice the celery with cucumber and pepper. Squeeze the soaked bread and puree it together with the tomatoes, garlic, salt, sugar, pepper and water with a hand blender. Mix the remaining vegetables with the pureed tomatoes and season with salt, sugar, pepper, vinegar and basil.

Gazpacho is a traditional Andalusian soup and is served as cold soup on hot days.

7.7.2 Asparagus Fennel Salad

You need:

A tuber of fennel, 30 asparagus spears, 2 avocado, juice and peel of a lemon, two tablespoons of linseed oil, salt, pepper, two tomatoes.

And here we go:

Brush the fennel in water and clean it. Cut the avocado in half, remove the seeds and cut into cubes of approx. 2cm thickness. Peel the asparagus. With the help of an Asian slicer, slice fine strips and do the same with the fennel bulb. Wash the tomatoes and cut into fine cubes. Mix all ingredients in a large bowl. Season to taste with salt, pepper, sugar and lemon juice as well as linseed oil and leave to stand for 1 hour. Serve cold. Linseed oil seeds have a high content of alpha linolenic acid, which is one of the omega 3 fatty acids. These have an anti-inflammatory effect and regulate blood lipids which in turn can have a positive effect on thrombosis, strokes and heart attacks.

7.7.3 Chiapudding

You need:

15 tablespoons chia seeds, 500g water, a teaspoon of cocoa, 20g sunflower seeds, 200g blueberries, two tablespoons honey.

And here we go:

Let the chia seeds soak in water overnight. Mix the berries together with the honey using a hand blender to make a puree. Roast sunflower seeds without fat in a pan. In tall glasses, first spread the chia seeds and then the berries. Garnish with cocoa and sunflower seeds.

Chia is a pseudo grain that was cultivated by the Mayas and Aztecs. The fruits of this ornamental plant come from Central America. Chia seeds are considered extremely healthy and can be used in smoothie, soup or salad.

7.8 Smoothie

Smoothie usually have a high nutrient density and may be full of carbohydrates in the form of fructose. Therefore, you should not consume these drinks regularly and in large quantities. If you need to mix for more than 90 seconds, add ice cubes or cold water to prevent the drinks from heating up and losing ingredients. Fibrous leaf green is often used in the recipes. If your blender reaches its limits, you can replace the ingredients with baby spinach, lamb's lettuce or lettuce. Also negative: Smoothie offers nothing to chew and is therefore detrimental to dental health.

Green smoothies contain mainly vegetables, sticks full of vitamins, secondary plant compounds, minerals and amino acids and are therefore preferable to fruit smoothies.

7.8.1 Chinese Cabbage Blueberry Smoothie

You need:

80g blueberries, one orange, one banana, 100g water, four medium sized leaves of Chinese cabbage

And here we go:

Remove the peel from the orange and banana and puree all ingredients with a high-speed mixer until creamy. Blueberries contain a lot of water and are low in calories. The proportion of provitamin A as well as vitamin C is high and is said to prevent cell damage. Main ingredients of Chinese Cabbage.

In addition to anthocyanins, vitamins and minerals, special tanning agents also make blueberries healthy. Tanning agents act against diarrhoea, inhibit the reproduction of bacteria and accelerate the healing of mucous membrane inflammations. However, this effect is observed especially in dried blueberries.

7.8.2 Green Detox Smoothie

You need:

140g kale, two, a piece of apple, half a banana, a cucumber, juice and peel of half a lemon, 240g water, a teaspoon of wheatgrass powder.

And here we go:

Wash the kale thoroughly. Then spin dry using a salad spinner. Do not peel the cucumber, just clean it in water with a vegetable brush. Cut it in half lengthwise and remove the seeds. Do not peel the apple, just remove the core. Cut the apple into small pieces. Mix all ingredients in a high-speed mixer to a creamy drink.

Wheatgrass powder belongs to the Super Foods and is said to strengthen the immune system and have a positive effect on the eyesight.

Kale stimulates digestion and helps us lose weight. It contains valuable fibre, which is important for our intestines and for good digestion. In addition, kale keeps us full longer due to the dietary fibres and prevents ravenous appetite attacks, as it keeps the blood sugar level constant.

7.8.3 Sauerkraut Grapefruit Smoothie

You need:

Half a grapefruit, 100g sauerkraut, half a pear, half an apple, a teaspoon of nut oil.

And here we go:

Halve the grapefruit and remove the skin. Blend all ingredients together with 100g water and a hand blender.

Sauerkraut with its lactic acid bacteria will make your digestion go faster. The pectin contained in the peel of pear and apple activates the bladder and kidney function. The grapefruit masked the taste of the sauerkraut. The nut oil contributes to the taste and ensures that fat-soluble vitamins can be absorbed by the body.

The grapefruit offers minerals such as potassium, calcium, magnesium, iron and phosphate. The plant substance naringin is responsible for the bitter taste of the fruit.

7.8.4 Avocado Banana Apple Smoothie

You need:

A handful of spinach, a boskop apple, a medium-sized banana, the flesh of a quarter avocado, the juice of an orange, 20g of ginger, 200g of water.

And here we go:

Wash and clean all components. Do not peel the apple, just remove the core. Blend all ingredients in a fast running mixer to a creamy drink. If necessary, increase the amount of water. Avocados are rich in unsaturated fatty acids and have a fat content of up to 30%. They are rich in minerals, especially magnesium, potassium and iron.

7.8.5 Chick peas smoothie, Greek yoghurt and broccoli

You need:

140g Greek yoghurt, a tablespoon of almonds, 70g broccoli, 70g strawberries, 30g chickpeas, 180g cold green tea, a quarter teaspoon of cinnamon.

And here we go:

Roast the almonds briefly in a pan without fat. Wash the strawberries and remove the green. Wash and dry the broccoli. Blend all ingredients together in a fast rotating mixer until creamy. Green tea contains plenty of caffeine and provides the necessary boost when consumed in the morning. Good for losing weight.

Broccoli contains a high dose of vital substances. These include vitamin B complexes as well as vitamins C, E and K; the minerals calcium, magnesium, iron, zinc and potassium and a large number of secondary plant substances that have a strong antioxidant effect.

7.8.6 Spinach Savoy cabbage smoothie with pear

You need:

80g fresh savoy cabbage, 80g baby spinach, two untreated pears, an apple, if possible boskop, half a bunch of mint, one tablespoon honey.

And here we go:

Savoy cabbage and apples clean remove the core. Wash and coarsely chop the savoy cabbage. Clean the baby spinach. Puree all ingredients together with 400g water in a suitable container using a hand blender.

Savoy cabbage contains glucosinolates. These sulphur-containing molecules give it its strong, spicy aroma and protect the cabbage from predators in nature. In the human body they can have an antioxidant effect.

7.8.7 Ginger Grape Carrots Smoothie

You need:

240g carrots, 90g seedless red grapes, 20g fresh ginger, one tablespoon rapeseed oil, 50g mineral water.

And here we go:
Remove the green at the end of the carrots. Brush under water, grate roughly with the skin. Clean the ginger. Blend all other ingredients in a blender or hand blender. The oil once again ensures that the fat-soluble vitamins are absorbed by the body. Ginger has an anti-inflammatory effect. Red grapes have a high content of B vitamins.

Ginger contains essential oils and gingerol, which gives it its pungency. In addition, the small tuber contains digestive and circulation stimulating substances such as Borneol and Cineol. Vitamin C, iron, magnesium, calcium, potassium, phosphorus and sodium are also contained. Ginger is therefore not only a tasty food, but also a remedy.

7.8.8 Pineapple Mango Detox Smoothie
You need:
An orange, 180g coconut water, half a mango, ¼ pineapple, juice and peel of half a lime, some cayenne pepper.
And here we go:
Remove the peel from the orange. Halve the mango, remove the core and remove the flesh. Cut the pineapple into quarters and remove the flesh from the skin and stalk. Blend all ingredients together with a hand blender.

Add a pinch of salt to taste. Season to taste with a little cayenne pepper.

Just like tomatoes, watermelons, carrots or oranges, pineapple has a diuretic effect. This is due to the potassium—it drains. The fibre and the enzyme bromelain help the intestines to get rid of toxins better. In addition, it contains vitamin C.

7.9 Mediterranean

7.9.1 Grilled Bread

You need:

500g flour, salt, a cube of yeast, 3 tablespoons of olive oil, half a red onion, a bunch of parsley leaves, 160ml strained tomatoes, 20g pine nuts, half an organic lemon, pepper, a finely chopped clove of garlic.

And here we go:

Mix the flour, salt, yeast, 160ml of warm water and a tablespoon of olive oil and work into a homogenous dough. Peel onion and cut into fine cubes. Wash parsley, dry with kitchen paper and chop finely with a sharp knife. Mix tomato sauce, onions, parsley, pine nuts, lemon juice and grated parsley and season to taste with salt, pepper and garlic. Roll out the dough on a work surface to a height of approx. 3cm and cut into three equally long strips. Weave the plait and spread the tomato sauce on top. Place in a warm place for another 20 minutes. Preheat the oven to 180° and bake the Mediterranean Grill Plait for about 25 minutes.

7.9.2 Fried fillet of gilthead

You need:

750g triplets, salt, pepper, 30g chopped garlic, ½ bunch of leaf parsley, 20g small capers, 230g cherry tomatoes, 1 bunch of rocket salad, 60g olive oil, 30g white wine vinegar, 20g liquid honey, four gilthead fillets, 20g butter, ½ lemon.

And here we go:
Wash and halve the potatoes. Then cook in salted water for about 8 minutes until al dente. Peel garlic and chop finely. Wash parsley, dry on a kitchen roll and chop finely. Drain the capers. Wash the tomatoes, remove the greens and cut them in half, wash the arugula, dry it and chop it finely. Heat oil in a pan and fry the potatoes in it. After about 4 minutes, add the tomatoes, vinegar, honey, garlic, parsley and capers and cook for another 2 minutes. Season to taste with salt and pepper. Rinse fish fillets cold and dry on a kitchen roll. Season with salt and pepper. Heat olive oil in a frying pan. Fry the dorade fillets on the skin side for about 3 minutes until it's crispy. Turn the fish fillets just before the cooking point, add the butter and fry for another 2 minutes over a low heat. Drizzle with lemon juice. Arrange the hot tomato potatoes on a plate. Place the fish fillet on top.

Triplets, also called small grading or field ware, are potatoes of a special size grading, regardless of the potato variety.

7.9.3 Anti Pasti with vegetables, mushrooms and olives

You need:

One aubergine, one zucchini, one green pepper, one yellow pepper, one red pepper, 200g of brown mushrooms, a bunch of leaf parsley, 150g of pitted green olives, 200g of olive oil, four cloves of garlic. Salt, pepper, 150g sugar, 150g Aceto Balsamico dark.

And here we go:

Wash and clean all the vegetables and cut them into strips about 2cm wide. Do not wash the mushrooms, but brush them. Wash the parsley leaves, dab dry and chop coarsely. Clean the garlic and mix it with the salt to a garlic paste. The following procedure is an example of the zucchini. Heat olive oil in a pan. Sauté the zucchini. Season with salt, pepper and garlic paste. Deglaze with 4cl Aceto Balsamico, add two tablespoons of sugar. Simmer for another 20 seconds, then remove from heat and leave to cool in the marinade. Do the same with the remaining vegetables. Cool overnight and season with salt and pepper the next day. Arrange everything together with the olives on a starter plate.

7.9.4 Penne in tuna tomato sauce

You need:

500g panicles of tomatoes, a clove of garlic, half a bunch of spring onions, a small medium hot red chilli, half a pot of basil, 120 g tuna in oil, salt, pepper, 50g olive oil, two shallots, 200g penne pasta.

And here we go:

Clean garlic and dice finely. Clean shallots and cut into cubes. Do the same with the spring onion. Clean the chillies and dice them finely. Wash the tomatoes, remove the greens and dice finely. Heat olive oil, sauté shallots and garlic briefly in it. Add spring onion and diced tomatoes. Season with salt, pepper and basil. Let simmer at mild heat for about 30 minutes. Drain the tuna and add to the tomato sauce. Cook penne noodles according to instructions. Arrange everything together on plates.

7.9.5 Pasta salad with mozzarella

You need:

400g spiral noodles, 200g tomatoes, 100 g rocket, 125g buffalo mozzarella, half a bunch of chives, 60g quark, 140g yoghurt, two tablespoons olive oil, two tablespoons white wine vinegar, pepper, salt, a clove of garlic.

And here we go:

Clean and chop the garlic. Clean and chop the chives. Cut mozzarella into large pieces. Cut tomatoes in half and mix with salt, sugar, pepper and olive oil. Mix curd cheese, yoghurt, olive oil, vinegar, salt and pepper to a salad dressing. Cook the spiral noodles in plenty of salted water, rinse cold. Mix with cherry tomatoes, rocket and mozzarella and garnish with chives.

7.9.6 Braised meatballs

You need:

280g green beans, 490g small potatoes, 60g pine nuts, 100g tomatoes, ½ bunch of thyme, 460g mixed mince, 45g breadcrumbs, 1 egg, salt, pepper, one red and yellow pepper, one medium red onion, 60g olive oil, 60 g tomato paste, 1 teaspoon vegetable stock (instant).

And here we go:

Wash and peel the potatoes and cook them in slightly salted water for about 5 minutes until al dente. In the meantime, clean and wash the beans. Add the beans to the potatoes and cook for another 8 minutes. Roast the pine nuts in a hot pan without fat. Wash the tomatoes, remove the greens and cut them into small pieces. Clean the thyme and chop finely. Chop the pine nuts. Mix the minced meat, breadcrumbs, egg, thyme, pine nuts and tomatoes. Season with salt and pepper. Form approx. six meatballs from the resulting mixture. Wash and clean the peppers, remove the core and cut into pieces. Peel onions and cut into strips. Fry the meatballs in hot fat for about 3 minutes on each side, remove and put aside. Lightly fry the bell peppers and the onions. Add tomato paste and cook for another 2 minutes. Deglaze with ¼ litres of water. Add broth, potatoes and beans and braise for another 4 minutes. Add the meatballs and cook for about 6 minutes.

7.10 Snacks

7.10.1 Leek Paprika Muffin

You need:

Two spring onions, a red pepper, a clove of garlic, two tablespoons of olive oil, half a bunch of basil, an egg, 50ml milk, 150g curd cheese lean step, salt, pepper, 40g grated Emmental cheese, 190g wholemeal spelt flour, a sachet of baking powder, a teaspoon of baking soda.

And here we go:

Clean the spring onion, peppers and garlic and cut into cubes of about 2cm. Heat the olive oil and steam the vegetables for about 5 minutes. Season with salt and pepper. In a bowl mix quark, milk, egg, Emmental, wholemeal spelt flour, baking powder and baking soda. Spread the mixture evenly in muffin cups and bake in a preheated oven at 180° for about 30 minutes. Muffins can be combined with vegetable dips or a crisp salad.

Leeks are one of the few foods with a high inulin content. Inulin is a soluble dietary fibre with extremely beneficial effects on the intestinal flora, which is why inulin is often taken as a food supplement as part of a healthy intestinal flora build-up.

7.10.2 Arancini-Sicilian rice balls

You need:

120g risotto rice, 60g frozen peas, salt, pepper, 40g flour, 60g breadcrumbs, one egg, 45 g boiled ham, 20g olive oil, 500ml vegetable stock, 70g grated Parmesan, two shallots. 500ml rape seed oil.

And here we go:

Finely dice boiled ham. Defrost the peas. Clean and dice the shallots. Heat olive oil, sauté shallots in it, add risotto rice. Cook the rice while stirring constantly. Add grated parmesan. Let the mixture cool down. Add flour, peas and boiled ham to the risotto mixture and mix. Form evenly sized balls. Heat rape oil. Turn the rice balls into the breadcrumbs and bake in hot rape seed oil. Drain on kitchen paper and let cool down.

Arancini are fried and felt rice balls. They are part of the traditional Sicilian cuisine and, depending on the province, they are conically shaped or filled with cheese or other vegetables.

7.10.3 Spinach Crostini au gratin

You need:

150g cream cheese, a medium sized shallot, 100g grated mountain cheese, 30g pine nuts, salt, pepper, 20g olive oil, two cloves of garlic, 110g leaf spinach, 300g ciabatta bread.

And here we go:

Sort and wash the spinach. Roast pine nuts in a pan without fat. Clean and chop the shallot. Heat olive oil and sauté the diced shallots. Add cream cheese and spinach. Heat up for 2 minutes. Finally add the mountain cheese. Stir until the mountain cheese has melted. Let the mixture cool down. Cut the ciabatta bread into 2cm thick slices and fry in a pan with olive oil. Spread the spinach mixture evenly on top and gratinate over the top.

Spinach contains a lot of vitamin C. This reduces the effect of the oxalic acid contained in green vegetables.

7.11 Vegan dishes

7.11.1 Pak Choi with ginger-garlic sauce and sesame

You need:

750g Pak Choi, two bunches of spring onions, 20g ginger, two cloves of garlic, three dried chillies, 40g rapeseed oil, 15g sugar, salt, pepper, 30g soy sauce, 20g dark balsamic vinegar, 5g cornflour, 50g white sesame seeds, 300g brown rice, 200g vegetable stock.

And here we go:

Clean and finely chop the spring onions, ginger, garlic and chillies. Heat 20g rapeseed oil in a frying pan and lightly sauté the previously cut vegetables for 2 minutes. Then top up with soy sauce, vinegar and 150g water. Mix cornflour with 30g water to thicken the above sauce. Lightly roast sesame seeds in a pan without fat. Pak Choi, clean, wash and divide into individual leaves. Cook the rice in lightly salted water. Sauté Pak Choi in 20g rapeseed oil colorless, add vegetable stock and steam covered for 3 minutes. Arrange the Pak Choi vegetables, pour the sauce over them and decorate with sesame seeds. Serve with brown natural rice.

Pak Choi has season from June to September. Strengthens the immune system, protects the body cells, does pregnant women good. It is also called Chinese mustard cabbage or Chinese leafy cabbage.

7.11.2 Baked aubergine, celery puree-carrots

You need:

200g celeriac, 2 tablespoons rapeseed oil, salt, one medium sized eggplant, 40g soy sauce, six carrots with green, oil for frying, 50g starch, pepper, sugar, 1 tablespoon light balsamic vinegar, 1 tablespoon agave syrup, 1 vanilla pod, 1 small red medium hot chilli pod.

And here we go:

Wash and clean the celery and cut into cubes. Lightly fry the cubes in 20g rapeseed oil, add a little water and season with a pinch of salt. Cover with a lid and cook until soft. Wash the aubergine, cut it into slices about 2cm thick and marinate with the soy sauce.

Brush the carrots, shorten the greens slightly and clean the carrot. Turn aubergine slices in the starch. Heat about 1 litre of fat to fry the aubergine in it. Halve the vanilla pod and remove the pulp. Cut the chilli pepper into small cubes.

Puree the celery in a blender and season to taste with light balsamic vinegar, salt, sugar and pepper. Heat the agave syrup and cook the carrots together with the diced chillies, vanilla pod and pulp in it.

7.11.3 Tomatoes stuffed with oriental couscous

You need:

200g couscous, 60g raisins, salt, pepper, 55g pine nuts, 1.5 tsp coriander seeds, ½ pot mint, 200g beef tomatoes, large, 2 tbsp olive oil, 1 tbsp of curry powder, hot. 20g rape oil.

And here we go:

Roast pine nuts in a pan without fat. Pour double the amount of hot water over the couscous and raisins and leave to stand. Coarsely crush coriander seeds in a mortar. Wash, dry and finely chop the mint. Wash the tomatoes, remove the green and cut in half. Remove the inside of the tomatoes and dice. Clean the garlic and chop finely. Mix the couscous with mint, coriander seeds, salt, pepper, finely chopped tomato cubes, garlic and the curry powder and fill into the tomato halves. Bake at 180 degrees in a preheated oven for about 30 minutes.

7.11.4 Bami Goreng with broccoli and tempeh

All ingredients are available in well-assorted Asian shops.

You need:

220g Mie noodles, 280g Tempeh, 140g pink mushrooms, 220g young wild broccoli, a bunch of spring onions, 40g rapeseed oil, 20g light soy sauce, 100g vegetable stock, 10g Sambal Olek, 30g roasted sesame seeds. For the marinade: a clove of garlic, 20g light soy sauce, 20g dark soy sauce, 10g maple syrup, 10g sesame oil.

And here we go:

Finely grate the clove of garlic and mix the remaining ingredients for the marinade. Cut the tempeh into 5 × 5 cm pieces and leave to stand in the garlic marinade for at least 1 hour. Cook the pasta in slightly salted water, drain and rinse with cold water. Fry the tempeh and the rest of the vegetables in rapeseed oil until colorless, deglaze with the vegetable stock, soy sauce and Sambal Olek. Add noodles, stir and season with salt. Serve and decorate with the roasted sesame seeds.

Tempeh is an important source of protein and comes from Asia. It is made from soybeans, just like tofu. Tempeh is inoculated with a noble mould and then fermented and stored for two days. This gives the product a slightly nutty taste. Available in the trade as a pressed product.

7.11.5 Sweet potato, chick peas and almond sauce
You need:

450g pre-cooked chickpeas, 10g ground cumin, 5g ground cinnamon, 5g ground coriander, 5g paprika powder, salt, pepper, 20g lime juice, 50g almond milk, sugar, half a bunch of chervil, 220g cherry tomatoes, 20g olive oil, 850g sweet potatoes, two cloves of garlic, 50g sesame paste

And here we go:

Peel sweet potatoes, cut into 2cm thick oblong slices, cut cherry tomatoes in half. Make a sauce from almond milk, lime juice, garlic and the sesame paste and put aside. Mix sweet potatoes and chick peas with all other ingredients. Preheat the oven to 180°. Line a baking tray with baking paper. Put marinated sweet potatoes and chick peas on the baking tray and cook for 50 minutes. After half the cooking time add the cherry tomatoes. Arrange sweet potato and chickpea tomato mix on plates, decorate with the sauce and chopped chervil.

7.11.6 Baked aubergine and carrots

You need:

200g celeriac, 2 tablespoons rapeseed oil, salt, one medium sized eggplant, 40g soy sauce, six carrots with green, oil for frying, 50g starch, pepper, sugar, 1 tablespoon light balsamic vinegar, 1 tablespoon agave syrup, 1 vanilla pod, 1 small red medium hot chilli pod.

And here we go:

Wash and clean the celery and cut into cubes. Lightly fry the cubes in 20g rapeseed oil, add a little water and season with a pinch of salt. Cover with a lid and cook until soft. Wash the aubergine, cut it into slices about 2cm thick and marinate with the soy sauce. Brush the carrots, shorten the greens slightly and clean the carrot. Turn aubergine slices in the starch. Heat about 1 litre of fat to fry the aubergine in it. Halve the vanilla pod and remove the pulp. Cut the chilli pepper into small cubes. Puree the celery with a blender and season with light balsamic vinegar, salt, sugar and pepper. Heat the agave syrup and cook the carrots together with the diced chillies, vanilla pod and pulp.

7.11.7 Zucchini Spaghetti | Lentil Bolognese

You need:

Three large courgettes, two large onions, 50g garlic, 150g carrots, 50g olive oil, 350 g pink lentils, 800 g tomatoes, 30g tomato paste, 10g oregano, salt, pepper.

And here we go:

Process the zucchini with a spiral slicer into pasta. Wash and peel the carrots and cut them into fine cubes. Do the same with onions, garlic and tomatoes. Lightly fry the sliced vegetables in olive oil and add tomatoes and tomato paste. Simmer for 2 minutes. Then add the pink lentils and pour in the vegetable stock. Cook covered for 15 minutes. Add oregano. Season to taste with salt and pepper. Heat olive oil in a frying pan, add the courgette pasta, season with salt and cook covered for 3 minutes. Bake

7.12 Bread

7.12.1 Best rye mixed bread without sourdough

You need:

345g wholemeal wheat flour type 550, 110g wholemeal rye flour, two teaspoons of salt, half a cube of fresh yeast, 360g water at room temperature.

And here we go:

Mix all ingredients in a large bowl and then cover. Let it rest for at least 16 hours, preferably in a warm, dark place. The dough should now have gained considerable volume. Carefully place the dough on a work surface and, without destroying its volume, carefully knead it again. Let the dough rest again for 2 hours, covered with a towel. Preheat the oven to 230° C. Put a bowl of water in the bottom of the oven. Place the dough on a baking tray lined with baking paper. If you have a cast-iron roaster with a lid, you can also use it. In this case, bake the first 20 minutes with the lid on, the rest of the time without the lid.

7.12.2 Whole grain spelt bread without rising

You need:

500g wholemeal spelt flour, approx. 120g grains of your choice, for example pumpkin seeds, sunflower seeds or walnut kernels, half a tablespoon of rock salt, half a litre of warm water, a cube of yeast, two tablespoons of apple vinegar.

And here we go:

Roast the grains in a pan without fat. Pour the warm water into a large bowl, mix the cube of yeast, salt and apple vinegar. Add the grains. Add the wholemeal spelt flour and mix well with a stirring spoon. Line a box form with baking paper. Add the bread dough. The oven does not need to be preheated. Then put the box form into the oven and bake at 190° C. Bake for 1 hour.

7.12.3 Foccacia

You need:

1 cube yeast fresh, 200ml lukewarm whole milk, 20g sugar, 70g pine nuts, 70g black olives pitted, 130g dried tomatoes pickled in oil, 500g flour type 405, salt, one egg, 3 tbsp tomato paste, 2 tsp dried oregano, 450g cherry tomatoes, 2 sprigs rosemary, coarse rock salt.

And here we go:

Mix lukewarm milk, yeast and sugar. Roast the pine nuts in a pan without fat. Let cool and chop. Cut the olives into quarters. Drain dried tomatoes and collect oil. Measure 100ml tomato oil and put aside. Dice the tomatoes. Mix the flour, pinch of salt and the yeast mixture. Add the oil, dried tomatoes and the egg. Knead to a smooth dough. Knead tomato paste, pine nuts, dried tomatoes, olives and oregano into the dough. Leave the dough to rise in a warm place, covered, for at least 2 hours. Preheat the oven to 180° C. Form the dough into a large flat cake and spread it flat on a baking paper. Press depressions into the dough. Wash and dry the tomatoes and spread the depressions. Wash, dry and pluck the rosemary and spread it on the dough. Sprinkle everything with rock salt and bake in the oven for about 30-35 minutes.

7.13 Sweet reward

7.13.1 Ricotta cheesecake-hazelnut caramel

You need:

700g ricotta, 110g maple syrup, one vanilla pod, 190g flour, 70g sugar, 125g butter, one teaspoon cocoa powder, two teaspoons gingerbread spice, one tablespoon cornflour, four eggs, one orange, a pinch of salt. 100g hazelnuts, 50g sugar, 80g water.

And here we go:

Knead cocoa powder, gingerbread spice, salt, flour, butter, brown sugar and form a dough ball. Store this dough ball in the refrigerator for about 30 minutes. Now bake the cake base blind. Cover a springform pan with baking paper. Roll out the dough on a work surface and line the edge of the springform pan about 3cm high. Cover this dough again with baking parchment, weight down with dry pulses and bake at approx. 180° for 15 minutes. For the mixture mix starch, vanilla pod pulp, maple syrup, ricotta, eggs, juice and orange peel. Pour this mixture onto the pre-baked base and bake at approx. 160° for 40 minutes.

For the hazelnut caramel, coarsely chop the hazelnuts in a mortar and boil them up with 80g water and the 50g sugar until the sugar caramelises.

7.13.2 Cheesecake Tiramisu in a glass

You need:

60 g butter, 120g lady fingers, 30g espresso powder (instant), 60g dark chocolate, 450g low-fat curd cheese, 550g mascarpone, 100g whipped cream, 170g sugar, 20g vanilla sugar, five eggs, 20g starch or custard powder.

And here we go:

Melt the butter. Hold back three pieces of the ladyfingers, crumble the rest. Mix the butter and crumbs, place them in six small ovenproof moulds and press them well onto the base. Preheat the oven to 150°. Make the cream. Mix the espresso, finely grated chocolate, quark, mascarpone, cream, sugar, vanilla sugar, eggs and starch to a smooth mixture. Pour this mixture into the six moulds, place in an appropriately sized pot and pour hot water up to 1cm below the rim. Cook in the oven for about 45 minutes. Let it cool down. Coarsely divide the remaining sponge fingers and sprinkle on the moulds.

7.13.3 Coffee Cream

You need:

300g milk, five leaves of white gelatine, three egg yolks, 30g sugar, 200g whipped cream, eight amarettini, cocoa powder, one vanilla pod.

And here we go:

Soak gelatine in cold water. Halve the vanilla pod and scrape out the pulp. Bring the pulp and pod to the boil with 250g milk and let it stand for a few minutes.

Mix the egg yolks together with the sugar in a bowl. Bring the milk to the boil again briefly and stir into the egg mixture. Stir constantly with a whisk. Squeeze the gelatine and add it to the hot mixture. Add the coffee powder. Chill the mixture and stir occasionally. Whip the cream until stiff. Just before the coffee cream starts to gel, carefully fold in the whipped cream. Then divide the mixture into four coffee cups and cool for at least 4 hours. Coarsely crumble the Amarettini. Process the remaining milk into milk foam. Decorate the coffee cream with the milk foam and the crumbled Amarettini.

7.13.4 Pear-Rhubarb Crumble

You need:

350g pears for example Williams Christ, 280g rhubarb, three tablespoons sugar, juice and grated lemon, one tablespoon vanilla custard powder, 40g almond biscuits, 30g butter, 30g oat flakes, two packs vanilla sugar.

And here we go:

Wash the pears, quarter them, remove the seeds and cut them into pieces. Clean the rhubarb and cut into 2cm thick pieces. Put the pears and rhubarb in a pot, add the sugar and lemon juice and bring to the boil covered. Mix the vanilla custard powder with two tablespoons of water to bind the pear-rhubarb mixture, bring to the boil and set aside. Pour the compote into small glasses.

Coarsely chop the almond biscuits with a knife. Melt the butter in a pan. Fry the oat flakes and almond biscuits in the pan until golden brown. Sprinkle with a little icing sugar and allow to caramelize. Put the cooled almond biscuits Oatmeal Crumble on the compote and serve.

7.13.5 Warm chocolate cake
You need:
110g dark chocolate, 70g butter, 50g sugar, a pinch of salt, two eggs, 20g flour.
And here we go:
Preheat the oven to 170 °C. Spread butter on four small ovenproof moulds and sprinkle with flour. Melt the chocolate in a hot water bath. Beat the soft butter, sugar and a pinch of salt in a bowl with a hand mixer until foamy. Add the eggs one by one and continue beating. Stir in the liquid chocolate. Add the flour and stir in with a wooden spoon. Fill the dough evenly into the moulds and bake in the oven for about 10 minutes. Serve the warm chocolate cake on a small plate, for example with a fruit sauce and sprinkle with icing sugar.

7.13.6 Semolina crème brulée with mango
You need:

Half a mango, 500g milk 3.5%, a pinch of salt, 60g sugar, the pulp of a vanilla pod, 50g wheat semolina, 40g brown sugar.

And here we go:

Halve a mango, remove the flesh and cut into cubes. Bring milk and sugar together with a pinch of salt to the boil. Add half of the mango to the mixture and puree everything using a blender. Stir in wheat semolina with a whisk. Let it swell for a short time and fill it into fireproof glasses while still warm. Spread the rest of the mango on the glasses, sprinkle with brown sugar and caramelise with a gas burner.

7.13.7 Vanilla-Ricotta cream with blueberries

You need:

250g ricotta, half a vanilla pod, juice of one lemon, 50g sugar, 250g blueberries, half a bunch of lemon balm, some icing sugar.

And here we go:

Put the ricotta in a bowl. Cut the vanilla pod lengthwise and scrape out the pulp. Add the vanilla pulp, juice and zest of one lemon, 50g sugar and a pinch of salt to the ricotta. Wash the blueberries. Pluck the lemon balm, add it to the blueberries with the icing sugar and mix.

Ricotta is an Italian cream cheese that can be made from sheep's or cow's milk. Translated this means „cooked again". Alternatively, cottage cheese can be used, which tastes as mild as ricotta. Also similar to ricotta is the Indian Panir cheese.

7.13.8 Carrots cup cake with walnuts

You need:

150g carrots, 150g walnuts, 50g wholemeal wheat flour, 140g sugar, three eggs.

And here we go:

Wash and peel the carrots. Grate finely on a kitchen grater. Separate yolks from whites. Add 100g sugar to the yolks. Then mix with a hand mixer until foamy. Beat the egg white with 40g sugar and a pinch of salt until stiff. Finely chop the walnuts. Carefully mix the egg yolks and the egg white mass together and fold in the walnuts, flour and carrots. Grease four fireproof baking dishes with butter and sprinkle with flour or breadcrumbs. Pour in the carrot mixture and bake at 180° for about 45 minutes. Sprinkle with icing sugar before serving.

7.13.9 Rhubarb Crumble

You need:

190g sugar, 90g butter, 610g rhubarb, a vanilla pod, juice and zest of one lemon, 70g oat flakes, 80g flour, one orange.

And here we go:

Mix oat flakes, a pinch of salt, flour and sugar. Add butter in small pieces and knead until small lumps are formed. Wash and clean the rhubarb and cut it into pieces about 2cm long. Halve the vanilla pod and scrape out the pulp. Wash the orange and remove the skin. Mix the rhubarb, sugar, lemon juice, vanilla pulp, orange peel and leave to stand for about 5 minutes. Pour the rhubarb mixture into a small casserole dish and spread the crumble over it. Bake in a preheated oven at 210° for approx. 40 minutes. A scoop of vanilla ice-cream would go perfectly with it. The whole thing means served.

7.13.10 Low Carb cream cheese pancakes

You need:

35g cream cheese, one egg, 50g almond flour, a teaspoon of xylitol, a pinch of salt, a teaspoon of coconut oil, 60g almond milk.

And here we go:

Mix all ingredients in a suitable container. The dough should not be too thick. Add some of the almond milk. Put the pancakes in a pan with a little oil as usual, until golden. Goes well with berries or vanilla ice cream.

Xylitol (chemically pentanentol) belongs to the group of sugar alcohols and is used, for example, in dental care chewing gums. Xylitol is similar in taste to normal household sugar, has almost the same sweetening power, but only one third of the calories. Almond flour can be used similarly to wholemeal wheat flour, but the amount of calories is reduced by about 53%.

8. List of recipes

9. Conclusion of Anti-inflammatory nutrition

You now know some of the most important background information that can contribute to the development of inflammation. Chronic diseases are on the rise in the western industrial nations. You now know that inflammations affect the whole body and can cause or trigger serious health problems.

The longer an inflammation lasts, the more clearly the immune defence is weakened and the more acidic our body becomes. Every inflammation should be taken seriously and acted upon accordingly. In order to act as quickly as possible if an inflammatory process is suspected, an experienced therapist or doctor should be consulted immediately. Unfavorable living habits and typical dietary mistakes are considered as accelerants of fire.

In order to take preventive action here, a preventive healthy anti-inflammatory lifestyle and diet is essential. I have shown you in this book how this can be achieved.

10. Feedback

I'm glad to hear your feedback. Did you like the book? Then I would be very happy about an honest evaluation. Just click on the following link.

https://amzn.to/3jX9vNU

Didn't you like the book? Even then I am happy about every feedback. Honest feedback is important to improve myself. If you have any suggestions or ideas for improvement I would be happy to hear from you. You can send any kind of request to the following e-mail address: book_manufacture@outlook.com.

Thanks for your support!

Best regards
Liam Wade

11. Sources

1 https://www.sciencedirect.com/topics/immunology-and-micro-biology/ethoxyquin

2 https://www.webmd.com/arthritis/about-inflammation

3 https://www.ncbi.nlm.nih.gov/pmc/articles/PMC2952901/

4 https://my.clevelandclinic.org/health/diagnostics/17747-sed-rate-erythrocyte-sedimentation-rate-or-esr-test

5 https://www.webmd.com/diet/anti-inflammatory-diet-road-to-good-health#1

6 https://www.ncbi.nlm.nih.gov/pmc/articles/PMC3614697/

7 https://en.wikipedia.org/wiki/Omega-3_fatty_acid

8 https://www.webmd.com/diet/anti-inflammatory-diet-road-to-good-health#1

9 https://medlineplus.gov/metabolicsyndrome.html

10 https://www.healthline.com/nutrition/why-trans-fats-are-bad

11 https://www.medicalnewstoday.com/articles/326941#causes

12. Copyright

All contents of this work as well as information, strategies and tips are protected by copyright. All rights are reserved. Any reprint or reproduction—even in part—in any form such as photocopying or similar processes, saving, processing, copying and distribution by means of electronic systems of any kind (in whole or in part) is strictly prohibited without the express written permission of the author.

All translation rights reserved. The contents of this book may under no circumstances be published. In case of disregard the author reserve the right to take legal action.

13. Disclaimer

The implementation of all information, instructions and strategies contained in this book is at your own risk and peril. They cannot replace consultation with a doctor. They are not medical advice. The author cannot accept liability for any damages of any kind for any legal reason. Liability claims against the author for material or non-material damage caused by the use or non-use of the information or by the use of incorrect and/or incomplete information are excluded in principle. Any legal and compensation claims are therefore excluded. This work has been compiled and written down with the greatest care and to the best of our knowledge and belief. However, the author accepts no responsibility for the topicality, completeness and quality of the information. Printing errors and misinformation cannot be completely excluded. No legal responsibility or liability of any kind can be assumed for incorrect information provided by the author.

14. Liability for links

My Books contains links to external websites of third parties, on whose contents we have no influence. Therefore I cannot take any responsibility for these external contents. The respective provider or operator of the sites is always responsible for the contents of the linked sites. The linked pages were checked for possible legal violations at the time of linking. Illegal contents were not found at the time of linking.

A permanent control of the contents of the linked pages is not reasonable without concrete evidence of a violation of the law. If I become aware of any infringements, I will remove such links immediately.

15. Imprint